Chinese Medicine

Paul U. Unschuld

Translated from the German by Nigel Wiseman

Paradigm Publications   **1998**   **Brookline, Massachusetts**

Chinese Medicine

Paul U. Unschuld

Translated by Nigel Wiseman

Copyright © 1998 Paradigm Publications

Library of Congress Cataloging-in-Publication Data:

Unschuld, Paul U. (Paul Ulrich), 1943–.

   [Chinesische Medizin. English]

   Chinese medicine / Paul U. Unschuld; translated from the German by Nigel Wiseman.

       p.   cm.

   Includes bibliographical references and index.

   ISBN 0-912111-55-0 (pbk.)

   1. Medicine, Chinese. 2. Medicine, Chinese—Philosophy.

3. Medicine, Chinese—History.   I. Title.

   [DNLM: 1. Medicine, Chinese Traditional. 2. Medicine, Chinese

Traditional—history.   WZ 80.5.06 U59c 1998a]

R601.U56913   1998

610' .951—dc21

DNLM/DLC

for Library of Congress   98-15490

                                                                                      CIP

Library of Congress Number: 98-15490

International Standard Book Number (ISBN): 0-912111-55-0

Published by

Paradigm Publications

44 Linden Street

Brookline, Massachusetts 02146 USA

e-mail: info@paradigm-pubs.com

Printed in the United States of America

CONTENTS

DESIGNATION

Paradigm Publications is a participant in the Council of Oriental Medical Publishers and supports their effort to inform readers of how works in Chinese medicine are prepared.

Chinese Medicine is an English translation of an original German-language work compiled from the sources cited in the Bibliography.

TRANSLATOR'S FOREWORD

Many introductions to Chinese medicine have appeared in the English language. *Chinese Medicine* differs in that, although it is not a history book as such, it is the work of a historian and is written from a historian's point of view, explaining events against the background of the life of the times in China. Paul Unschuld's *Chinese Medicine* introduces each element of the Chinese medical corpus of knowledge; each phase of its development in the light of the intellectual, social, political, and economic soil from which it sprang.

As the author tells us, a medical system develops its theories, and gains and maintains the acceptance of the community it serves not by its clinical effectiveness but by the acceptability of its underlying ideas. From this perspective, *Chinese Medicine* explains how the concepts of Chinese medicine were able to gain acceptance, and how, despite its gradual evolution, its basic features remained stable for two thousand years. From the same perspective, it also explains the conditions that have allowed the survival of Chinese medicine into the modern age in China despite China's adoption of Western medicine as the mainstay of its health-care system; and the conditions in which, after centuries of European interest in and rejection of China's healing arts, Chinese medicine has finally taken root in the West. It is this dimension of *Chinese Medicine* that sets the book apart from others of its kind. Aside from the wealth of information it contains about the nature and development of Chinese medicine, the author's view of the reception of Chinese medicine in the West is a major contribution to our understanding of alternative health care, and forcefully challenges the conceptions of Chinese medicine among many of its Western adherents.

This is one of Paul Unschuld's more slender volumes; despite its size, it is immensely informative, unapologetically objective, not to say delightfully controversial.

Taichung, March 1997   Nigel Wiseman

AUTHOR'S PREFACE

Traditional Chinese medicine is a multifaceted cultural heritage, which after a history of two thousand years in East Asia and after a 400-year period of transmission to the West, is now, at the end of the 20th century, overcoming its former exclusively regional significance to become a resource exploited in all industrial countries of the West.

The present work explains the features of Chinese medicine and the causes of and circumstances surrounding its introduction into Europe as well as the problems of its integration into our health system.

We do not attempt to provide a history of Chinese medicine from its beginnings up to the present any more than we attempt to give a general presentation of this form of healing in all its many facets of theory and practice.

The perspective chosen is historical only insofar as it calls for comparison of the past and present of Chinese medicine, as well as occasionally of certain features of Chinese and Western medicine. The aim of the discussion is to highlight the basic elements of Chinese medicine in the field of tension between its historical birth in East Asia and its new interpretation and application in China and the West.

Munich, May 1997   Paul U. Unschuld

CHAPTER ONE
INTRODUCTION

In 1972, Richard Nixon visited the People's Republic of China in a spectacular reorientation of US policy on East Asia. Western journalists following the US President on their return reported in detail about the Chinese alternative to the socioeconomic realities in other countries of the Communist Bloc and the Third World. Maoist groups formed in all Western countries and propagated the Chinese way toward a "new" society as a generally applicable solution, which, they claimed, also promised success in dealing with the problems of highly industrialized countries.

In this context, interest focused not only on Chinese achievements apparently worthy of emulation such as collective management of industry and public self-criticism of individual failings, but also on some most astounding Chinese healing practices, which allegedly sprang from the experience of the people, and, as it appeared to many, were conducive to bringing the medicine of the bourgeois establishment back to a popular line. So-called barefoot doctors and acupuncture, in particular acupuncture anesthesia, were presented by the Western media to a marveling public as the quintessence of Chinese medicine and as a serviceable alternative to progressively professionalized and medicalized health care. With this began a development whose effects on the practice of medicine in Europe and the USA are still visible today, over two decades later.

Attempts to use needles instead of drugs to achieve anesthesia even in major surgical operations have in the meantime slipped into deserved oblivion, just as much as collective management and public self-criticism. It was not until after the "Great Proletarian Cultural Revolution" in 1976 and the opening of China in 1978 that Chinese doctors were able to report, without personal risk, about the pain that patients had been expected to endure through therapy applied in operating theaters not on the basis of scientific knowledge, but in accordance with the ideological precepts of the Communist Party.

Nonetheless, since that time, acupuncture has gained influence in Europe and the USA, and its pain-relieving abilities are widely recognized today; in actual fact, acupuncture is now probably the most significant non-drug therapy used around the world to relieve or completely eliminate pain of various origins. A no longer negligible number of doctors and healers are applying acupuncture outside Asia in all European countries, as well as in the USA, Australia, and New Zealand. In this way, a part of traditional Chinese healing practices has found recognition in societies in which, until a few years ago, Western medicine, committed to Western science and rationality, appeared to possess an irrevocable monopoly with regard to the explanation and treatment of sickness.

This development has been associated with some widespread misunderstandings. Acupuncture has been and still is frequently equated with Chinese medicine. It is only over the last few years that particularly in the USA traditional Chinese drug therapy, which is a central component of traditional Chinese medicine, has been accorded greater attention. In Germany, only initial attempts have been made to apply Chinese drug therapy because of German legislation and possibly because European herbalism has not completely died out there.

A further misunderstanding has been to equate China and "the Chinese" with reverence and use of Chinese medicine. In actual fact, Chinese medicine has been on the defensive in its homeland for a century. With some exaggeration, we might say that the significance of acupuncture and traditional drug therapy has waned in China as much as it has grown in Europe and the USA. Such vicissitudes of a system of medical ideas and practices have little to do with their actual clinical effects, and depend—

as I will try to show—on the power of conviction that the ideas underlying a healing system exert on a population.

Finally, yet another misunderstanding should also be pointed out. A widely-held view is that traditional Chinese medicine as applied in the industrialized countries of the West is a perfect reflection of the traditional Chinese medicine that is currently practiced in China, and that this in turn is a true reflection of traditional Chinese medicine as practiced in China for two millennia or more. In such a view, this millennia-old Chinese medicine has since time immemorial constituted a complete alternative to Western medicine as if both were as diametrically opposed as sun and moon or fire and water.

In fact, the Chinese medicine that patients in Europe and the USA are turning to is not to be compared with the reality of the healing system in East Asia, and the various very different manifestations of Chinese medicine in China, Japan, and other Asian countries are all likewise removed from the historical reality before the 20th century.

The notion of a vast dichotomy between Western and Chinese reactions to disease is completely unfounded. Seen against its historical background, what is now very much an "alternative" Chinese medicine is only a minimal vestige of ideas and practices that, having been extracted from a highly impressive variety of medical thought, and supplemented with modern elements of Western rationality, was only recently placed in artificial opposition to Western approaches. In its basic theoretical features, which since the Hàn Dynasty two thousand years ago have been described in writing in all their details, traditional Chinese medicine is quite closely related to the explanations of physical and mental suffering that developed in Europe and to the notions of appropriate responses to sickness that derived from them. Only in modern times have the traditions of the East and West of a huge common continent been brought into an unfounded opposition.

Large parts of everyday life in China now bear the imprint of Western culture, Western science, and Western technology. Nevertheless, it would be premature to believe that this development will mean the end of Chinese culture as an independent entity. Chinese music, traditional Chinese dress, and traditional architecture, as well as many other elements of the old culture, may survive as parts of the scenery on the otherwise modernized stage of Chinese life. This circumstance, however, should not blind us to the fact that China has also carried over from its past into its present certain approaches to knowledge and to the body that are perhaps only temporarily or seemingly subordinated to Western rationality.

Signs are already visible in China as well as in Japan that these two East-Asian cultures and the West are interacting and amalgamating in various ways. By contrast, the West, proudly conscious of the scientific and technological superiority that it has enjoyed so far, is rooted solely in its own ways of thought. Whether the nations of the Far East will gain some advantage from knowledge of their own and foreign traditions is a moot point, but is not to be completely dismissed out of hand. For this reason, it might at some point prove meaningful to provide, for example, Chinese medical knowledge of past centuries with a sober evaluation from a Western perspective.

If we look at the current reality of especially Europe and the USA, we see that not too much is going on in this respect. Hundreds, if not thousands, of historians, philosophers, and theoreticians of knowledge are studying the history of European science since Aristotle. Only a handful of mostly young enthusiasts are attempting to penetrate the traditions of Chinese mathematics, physics, and botany. There is no university-affiliated institute in the West equipped to support serious long-term systematic research. Sinologists attempting to deal with these questions have to seek their livelihood outside their discipline.

Traditional Chinese medicine is no exception. Although there is widespread interest in clinical applications, serious research into the content and dynamic of this part of Chinese culture occurs mostly only sporadically, outside the realm of sinology. This makes one ponder, for no field is better suited to understanding a foreign culture as medicine. Here, natural history and philosophy, ethics and religion, language and literature, society and economy, technology and handicraft meet together. The study of Chinese medicine permits a view of Chinese culture that can make an essential contribution to understanding the historical and present dimensions of a far-away exotic land that modern communications and transportation have now turned into a frequently visited partner country in trade and politics.

Chapter Two
The Early Formative Phase

1. A new world view

In European antiquity, the formation of a body of medical thought around 500 B.C., though precisely datable in time, was a cultural achievement that coincided with the beginning of literary culture, and for this reason can be contrasted with the background of older notions of healing only to a limited extent. In China, on the other hand, a comparable expansion of a world view characterized by gods, demons, and ancestors to embrace the laws of nature in the 3rd to the 2nd centuries B.C., and the subsequent development of a medicine based purely on natural laws in the 2nd and 1st centuries before Christ, came at a time when there were already numerous writings, some of which are still extant today, providing information about older layers of thought.

Evidently only one or two centuries behind Greece, Chinese thinkers in the second half of the first century B.C. perceived the possibility of discovering the "Way," that is, laws apparent in nature and in the social life of human beings, recognition of which provides the key to self-determination. Belief in the existence of gods and spirits that could intervene in human life was lost neither in the East nor in the West of the Eurasian continent, yet it would appear that Chinese society drew generally more consistent conclusions from the perception of natural laws than did European society.

Together with the realization of being a part of a natural, integrated whole constituted by the microcosm and macrocosm that was valid in its own right, there developed a rather distanced approach to matters metaphysical and, for part of the population, the once flourishing and emotionally laden encounter with the numinous aspect of life froze into a cold ritual. "The Way knows neither demons nor spirits, it comes of itself and goes of itself," as succinctly stated in *The Inner Canon of the Yellow Thearch* (黄帝内经 *huáng dì nèi jīng*), the classic of the tradition of medicine oriented towards natural laws that started to be compiled in the first century B.C.

This process was still not fully completed in the second century B.C. In the items accompanying a noble couple and their son in the Mǎwángduī (马王堆) tomb in Chángshā in the Province of Húnán, which was sealed in 167 B.C., there are clear signs of the new mode of thinking alongside the old traditions in an upper stratum of the population. In the total of 15 medical texts, which were buried alongside other items of an evidently comprehensively equipped home for the afterlife of its occupants, magical and demonological material is found side by side with prescriptions that attest a surprisingly sophisticated knowledge of pharmacy and new notions of the significance of blood vessels for health and life.

Findings from a tomb in Zhāngjiāshān (张家山) in Húběi Province dating from the 2nd century B.C., from a tomb in Shuānggǔduī (双谷堆) in Ānhuī Province of the year 165 B.C., as well as a tomb in Shuìhǔdì (睡虎地), again in Húběi Province, dating from the year 217 B.C., complete our picture of a multi-faceted revolution in the understanding of disease.

Knowledge of the power of ancestral spirits to endanger or even destroy human life had existed since prehistoric times. For centuries, if not millennia, it appeared that these normally invisible cohabitants of the world could be pacified by an accommodating way of life aligned to certain norms, or, if they became wrathful, could be appeased by appropriate requests and sacrifices. In the middle of the first millennium B.C., the notion of demons that could be kept in check not by customs and morals (by the individual's own behaviour), but only by higher forces, came to the fore.

This belief that demons could cause disease and could cause harm in various other aspects of daily life has continued among some parts of the Chinese population into the present. Yet the world view of a majority of the educated élite since the Hàn period (206 B.C.–A.D. 220) has been oriented not toward the incalculable but toward the calculable. Piece by piece, correspondences were uncovered that made the work of demons seem unlikely. The insight, for example, that a connection existed between the circumference of the moon and the tides of the sea, which Wáng Chōng (王充, A.D. 27-97) emphasized, largely silenced voices that had interpreted the ebb and flow as signs of the activity of spirits.

The texts recovered from tombs lead us into the variety of diverging views of the early Hàn period. This time appears very remote, but we might consider that it corresponds to the latter phase of Hellenism and the early phase of the Roman empire, and that it was characterized by an intellectual dynamic of equal rank. The broad geographical distribution of the sites of findings and the closeness and sometimes even literal agreement between the texts found gives some idea of the great distances over which thoughts and writings were being exchanged at the time and of the number of individuals involved in the revision of thought.

2. Disease as foe; therapy as battle

At that time, the two styles of thinking that have characterized Chinese medicine for over two thousand years until the present were consolidated. One was connected with the belief in demons. We call it "ontic" because it traces disease to intruders in the body or at least to damage inflicted on the body by evil beings outside. Numerous names refer to various demons capable of such deeds. Many strategies developed to evade demons or expel them from the body. The instigator was the disease, and it was among the tasks of the shamans (巫 wū) and the prescription experts (方士 fāng shì) to provide remedies through magic means.

According to general popular belief, the evil-bringing demons were not at all only invisible beings; they also appeared in tangible form, as a fox or human, but very often as an insect or worm. They could be chased away by the power of words, claims to allegiance with higher powers, the use of fire at the site of the suffering, or by trampling the things identified as demons under foot, such as a certain number of egg yolks when an illness affecting a whole family had been attributed to demons in the form of egg yolks.

The gradual loss of plausibility of such concepts and corresponding action among a section of the intellectual elite of the Hàn era led first of all to the inclusion of naturalistic concepts and finally to the dominance of an ontic, yet at the same time, purely empirical-pragmatic tradition of healing. The enemies to be repelled, driven out of the body, or killed were now not primarily demons, but environmental factors such as cold and heat, dampness and dryness, or bugs, or illness as an abstract, but nevertheless real, evil.

Chinese healers of pre-Hàn antiquity were acquainted with numerous forms of human suffering that took the same form in whomever they afflicted or at whatever time they occurred. These are called diseases. They exist independently of the afflicted individual and are referred to by set names that among the educated invoke identical conceptions of a particular kind of illness.

Many of the disease names of Chinese antiquity are no longer accessible to etymological interpretation. One example is the name nüè (疟) for malaria, whose origin will probably remain hidden forever.

Some disease names of course do offer room for thought about their origin. Many designations are derived from the supposed cause, as, for example, in the case of leprosy, which was known, amongst other things, as "míng disease" because míng (螟) bugs obviously ate not only grain, but could also destroy the features of the human face from inside the body.

When General Mǎ Yuán (14 B.C.–A.D. 49) returned from a campaign against insurgent people in the south, the Chinese learned about a new disease, the pox, which spread rapidly among the troops. Because of its origin, it was called *lǔ chuāng* (虏疮), "prisoners-of-war sores," and was later, on account of the bean-shaped pustules, called *dòu* (痘), "bean disease," a name by which the disease is still known to this day in China.

Other ancient disease names suggest a pathological process. One example is the name for diabetes; the Chinese term *xiāo kě* (消渴) literally means "flowing away and thirst." The earliest descriptions characterized this disease as the result of prolonged consumption of sweet and fatty foods. The first *xiāo kě* patient we know of was the famous poet Sīmǎ Xiàngrú (司马相如, died 117 B.C.).

Noteworthy about the designation *xiāo kě* is the fact that its conceptual context finds no explanation in ancient Chinese medicinal literature. However, in Aretaios of Cappadocia (1st century A.D.), diabetes is described as a disease in which the patient has a great *thirst* and drinks a lot, but voids still larger amounts of fluid and in this way *flows away*.

Equally surprising and open to conjecture are disease names that correspond in terms of their meaning and occasionally even in their pronunciation to specific terms used in Greek antiquity. In ancient texts, we find the designation *fèi xiāo* (肺消), "pulmonary wasting," which is a literal equivalent of the Greek term *phthisis*, both referring to pulmonary consumption. This coincidence is all the more remarkable insofar as ancient Chinese medicine, though it knew about the morphology of the internal organs, made no attempts to develop theoretical considerations of any pathological changes in these organs or of changes brought about elsewhere in the body by these organs. This would invite the conjecture that the notion of "pulmonary consumption" entered China from abroad.

Against this background, the term *huò luàn* (霍乱) also seems to be worthy of attention. Translated literally, this term means "swift and uncontrolled," and in ancient texts refers to violent vomiting accompanied by profuse diarrhea. The term *huò luàn* is still used to this day to denote cholera, and gives cause to wonder whether it is simply a Chinese transcription of the Greek equivalent.

Finally, one example of foreign influence outside the realm of disease should be mentioned. It may be a reasonable hypothesis that Qí Bó (岐伯), the most important interlocutor of the Yellow Thearch in the *Inner Canon of the Yellow Thearch*, is none other than Hippocrates. Qí Bó is a man who has no historical background in Chinese history or mythology, and this fact, together with the Hàn-period pronunciation of his name, allows speculation that the fame of the Greek physician reached China two centuries after his death.

Ancient Chinese disease names appear in many places in the historical records of the late Zhōu period (1122–255 B.C.). The focal text representing the attempt to provide a prescription for each and every disease is one of the Mǎwángduī texts from the early second century B.C., the *Wǔ Shí Èr Bìng Fāng* (五十二病方), in whose fragments 282 prescriptions for 52 diseases can be found. The structure of the individual entries generally obeys a strict causal thinking. The description of the symptoms of the disease is followed by a statement of the causes, this in turn by directions for therapy.

The *Wǔ Shí Èr Bìng Fāng* offers an exemplary combination of demonology and medicine; it is the recognizable starting point for the development of an increasingly varied prescription and materia medica literature over the following two thousand years. The fight in allegiance with metaphysical powers against demons was replaced by the fight in allegiance with medicinal drugs against disease. The motto "using drugs is like deploying soldiers" has accompanied Chinese pharmacy into the present and explains the military terminology widely prevalent in Chinese medicine.

3. The yīn-yáng doctrine

Magic is a putative natural law handed down from prehistoric times, whose effects are independent of gods and ghosts. In the narrow sense, magic derives from the perception that like things behave in like ways and that parts of a former whole remain a whole. These relationships have consequences for influencing natural processes.

An image or effigy is part of the original; what is inflicted on it is also inflicted on the original. A lock of hair or fingernail remains part of the individual from which it was taken. Whatever is done to it is also experienced by the person to whom it belongs. A walnut resembles the brain in appearance; the consumption of walnuts therefore strengthens the brain. The string of a crossbow represents the principle of acceleration; laid around the body of a woman in labor, it speeds delivery.

Possibly as a result of a common cause, in the middle of the first century B.C., attempts developed not only in the eastern Mediterranean but also—only a little later—in China to reduce the things and phenomena of the world to a limited number of groups of similar phenomena. The interrelationship between these groups supposedly followed certain laws, which provided the means to understand the relationship of any individual phenomenon to other phenomena within and outside the group to which it belongs.

The first comprehensive systematization of things and phenomena forms the second major way of thinking that characterized the Chinese understanding of nature for two thousand years until the encounter with the Western natural sciences. This, as we call it, "systematic" way of thinking made it possible not only to understand natural processes, but also to influence them. In medicine, as in other areas, these conceptions attained practical application.

Within this systematic way of thinking, two different approaches were applied in the grouping of all things and phenomena, both of which have continued to provide the theoretical basis of the traditional explanatory model of Chinese medicine up to the present.

In one approach, Chinese thinkers developed a dualistic scheme for the organization of things and phenomena, widespread among many cultures, into the complex and multilayered yīn-yáng doctrine. The heart of this doctrine rests on the insight that all things and phenomena have an opposite with which they form a unity. The two poles in unity were given the names yīn and yáng, which derived from the shady and sunny side of a hill.

From simple and obvious categorizations such as heaven, sun, day, and fire as yáng, and earth, night, moon, and water as yīn, adherents of the doctrine gradually incorporated more and more finely distinguished things and increasingly abstract phenomena, so that each phenomenon was, as it were, allotted its place in the system, and its nature and function could be understood and explained in terms of an all-embracing dynamic of birth, life, and death.

In pre-Hàn antiquity, the originally purely dualistic yīn-yáng doctrine had already undergone a fourfold and sixfold differentiation. Phenomena such as the seasons gave cause for the following groupings:

> Yáng in yáng or pure yáng (e.g., summer)
>
> Yīn in yáng or maturing yīn (e.g., autumn)
>
> Yīn in yīn or mature yīn (e.g., winter)
>
> Yáng in yīn or maturing yáng (e.g., spring)

Knowledge of a considerable number of organs of the body was incorporated into two groups each of three different yīn and yáng qualities:

> Major yīn (lung and spleen)
>
> Minor yīn (heart and kidneys)

Ceasing yīn (heart-enclosing network and liver)

Major yáng (small intestine and urinary bladder)

Yáng brilliance (large intestine and stomach)

Minor yáng (gallbladder and triple burner)

For the purposes of medicine, it was necessary and possible to categorize all organs and body parts, all physiological, etiological, and pathological processes, as well as therapeutic measures in the yīn-yáng groups and, starting from this, to select the appropriate response to those situations requiring treatment.

4. The doctrine of the five phases

The doctrine of the five phases arose from the same conceptions of an all-encompassing system of correspondence of things and phenomena as the doctrine of yīn and yáng. The origin of the significance of the number five is not known. On the oracle bones of the Shāng Dynasty (1766–1122 B.C.) we already find references to five directions: west, east, north, south, and center. From the middle of the first millennium B.C., six basic elements of human existence were identified: water, fire, metal, wood, earth, and grain. At the same time, numerous fivefold groupings of all things and phenomena such as colors, flavors, qualities of voice, and many others appeared in literature. Finally, a gradually developing fivefold categorization of all things and phenomena came to center around the five symbols water, fire, metal, wood, and earth.

In European secondary literature, the group symbols were for a long time erroneously translated as "five elements," evidently an adaptation to the four elements fire, water, earth, and air of Greek antiquity. The related notion that metal, wood, water, fire, and earth, like the four elements of Greece, were the basic building blocks out of which everything was made is evidenced in China by a single quotation: "Thus the kings of yore mixed earth with metal, wood, water, and fire, and created in this way the hundred things." This statement, however, stood in no recognizable philosophical context and did not form the basis of any corresponding system of thought.

Metal, wood, water, fire, and earth are five symbols that most appropriately explain reciprocal relationships and effects between things and phenomena that are classified by them into five groups. The translation "five evolutive phases" (fünf Wandelphasen) introduced by Richard Wilhelm (1873–1930) has given birth to the term "five phases," which reflects the dynamic of the model: things and phenomena do not exist statically beside one another, but affect each other, and in chronological sequence, after each other.

The relationships of overcoming (相克 *xiāng kè*), documented as early as the late Zhōu period, stand in the foreground.

> Wood overcomes earth
>
> Earth dams water
>
> Water extinguishes fire
>
> Fire melts metal
>
> Metal cuts wood

In the early Hàn period, engendering relationships (相生 *xiāng shēng*) appear:

> Wood engenders fire
>
> Fire engenders ashes/earth
>
> Earth engenders minerals/metals
>
> Out of water come minerals/metals
>
> Water engenders wood

The relationships of engendering and overcoming are found again in the controlling relationship:

> When metal cuts wood excessively, the son of
> wood, i.e., fire, comes to wood's assistance
> and melts metal
>
> When water extinguishes fire excessively, the
> son of fire, i.e., earth comes to fire's assis-
> tance and dams water
>
> When wood moves earth excessively, the son of
> earth, i.e., metal, comes to earth's assistance
> and cuts wood
>
> When fire melts metal excessively, the son of
> metal, i.e., water, comes to metal's assistance
> and extinguishes fire
>
> When finally water dams earth excessively, the
> son of water, i.e., wood, comes to water's as-
> sistance and moves earth

However plausible these and certain other relationships appear, it was not without difficulty that important phenomena not
least in the medical context were assigned to individual groups.

While one author thought it appropriate to assign the spleen
to the phase wood and hence to the color blue-green, the lung to
the phase fire and the color red, the heart to earth and yellow,
the liver to metal and white, and the kidney to water and black,
the author of another text thought it fitting to associate the
liver with blue-green, the heart with red, the spleen with yellow,
the lung with white, and the kidneys with black. If one author
assigned the spleen to sheep, the lung to hens, the heart to cattle,
the liver to dogs and the kidney to pigs, another text would
associate the liver with hens, the heart with sheep, the spleen
with cattle, the lung with horses, and the kidney with pigs.

So long as the Hàn Dynasty was associated with the earth
phase, the heart, which already in the Zhōu period had been
designated as the most important organ, was considered to belong to the earth phase. Yet with the beginning of the later Hàn
period, fire came to be identified with this dynasty, and from
that time, the heart was equated with fire.

Although until the early years of the Western Hàn, only four seasons were defined, consequently leaving one of the five phases without a season assigned to it, the season "late summer" (长夏 *cháng xià*) was discovered as the fifth season, thereby assuring the comprehensive validity of the system.

Over a period of one or two centuries, Chinese thinkers ordered and extended the arrangement of things and phenomena according to the five phases again and again, until finally, on the basis of criteria that are no longer clear, a scheme was found which was afterward occasionally called into question, but which remained the basis of the systematic way of thinking of the Chinese natural history and medicine without further change.

The dynamics of the five phases found its medical application among other things in the explanation of the transmission of disease-causing agencies in the organism, in diagnosis, in diet, in psychology, and over a thousand years later beginning in the 12th century, in the use of drugs.

For example, a patient who is excessively pensive can be treated by producing anger in him. Pensiveness is the emotion of the spleen and therefore the phase earth. Anger is the emotion of the liver and therefore of wood. Since wood can overcome earth, anger can put an end to pensiveness.

Another example of the application of five-phase theory in medicine may illustrate the role of the five phases in prognosis and treatment of disease. A pathogenic agent, which is transmitted from the liver to the spleen, is more threatening than one that reaches the lung from the liver since the liver belongs to the wood phase and overcomes the spleen, which belongs to earth. Conversely, the lung, i.e., the metal phase, generally represents no threat to the spleen, the earth phase.

For treatment, this means that two patients, in both of whom a disease of the liver has been established, must be treated differently once it is determined that the disease has entered the spleen from different sources. It is therefore important to know—

and this is a fine example for the close and almost inextricable connection between ontic and systematic thinking in Chinese medicine—where a disease-causing agency is at the point of treatment.

If, for example, evil cold has gained access into the body through the lung, it may stay there, or it may move on. The lung is assigned to metal. When metal is struck, it sounds. Whether the cold evil has stayed in the lung or has attacked other organs from there can be determined from the voice qualities ascribed to the various organs.

If an illness arose by wind being able to penetrate the body, the organ of entry is always the liver, since the liver, like wind, belongs to the evolutive phase wood and the season spring. Whether wind remains in the sphere of the liver or is conveyed in the organism to another functional sphere can be determined by the various colorations of the facial complexion, for spring is the time when color replaces the gray of winter, and it is logical that wind, which is part of the wood phase, is visible in the organism through the complexion.

In similar fashion, the theory of systematic correspondence suggests that changes in the odor of the breath and the body can be traced to diseases arising from alien heat in the body (since things thrown into a fire develop a characteristic smell), and that any change in the excretion of fluids such as tears or saliva is seen to be caused by diseases attributable to penetration of dampness into the organism.

Every major organ is associated with one of the five flavors. In certain pathological situations, it is appropriate to provide a major organ with the flavor with which it is associated—either in the form of food or in the form of drugs. Both foods and drugs are associated with at least one of the five flavors, and just as in magical correspondence walnuts strengthen the brain, so in the comprehensive system of correspondences between things, a sweet flavor strengthens the spleen, because both sweetness and the spleen belong to the earth phase.

5. The structure of the organ system

The initial unification of the Chinese empire by the first emperor of the Qín Dynasty (reigned 221–206) introduced a completely new state structure such as had never been known before in China. Different parts of the country grew together as they became linked through a system of roads and waterways. Harmonization of weights, measures, writing, and other things contributed to the integration of the lives of formerly separate political entities into a monolithic empire.

The body was viewed in a similar way. Individual organs had been known for a long time, just as individual vessels running through the body had been. Yet it was not until the late second or even the first century B.C. that these individual parts grew together producing an organism in which each organ was dependent on the others and contributed in various ways to supplying the needs of the body as a whole.

Five "depots" (藏 zàng), the lung, heart, spleen, liver, and kidney, and six "administration units" or "palaces" (府 fǔ), the small intestine, large intestine, stomach, gallbladder, urinary bladder, and triple burner, form the central functional units of the organism. In addition, a sixth depot, the heart-enclosing network, was identified, which was brought into play only when the application of the yīn-yáng doctrine called for a sixfold organization of the central organs. The brain, the marrow, and the uterus were discussed as organs, but for numerical reasons, they had no lasting recognition.

The Nàn Jīng (难经), "The Classic of Difficult Issues," an important text from the first century A.D., offered a detailed morphological and topographic description of the organism, from which we can infer that at some time relevant knowledge had developed through dissection or had been imported into China from outside. For reasons that cannot be explained, probing the internal terrain of the body remained uninteresting for China at least since antiquity. The knowledge that had accumulated in whatever way by this time remained the uncontested basis of the conceptions of the interior of the body and the processes occurring there.

At the center of Chinese conceptions of healthy and morbid processes in the organism stood a complex system of conduits (经络 *jīng luò*), which like the roads and waterways of the unified empire, penetrated the whole body and the limbs, as well as the depots and palaces, and thereby connected them. Twelve main conduits (经 *jīng*) were connected with network vessels (络 *luò*), which ramified further into tertiary vessels (孙络 *sūn luò*). In addition, there were special conduits outside the constant circulation that had a certain function as reservoirs.

The system of conduits and network vessels complemented an older conception of the blood vessels. For a long time, the blood vessels, visible under the skin, had evidently been a focus of diagnosis and treatment. Determining whether the veins were full or empty, and the skin covering them was smooth or rough, provided data about the state of the patient. Fullness was treated by bleeding, and emptiness by the application of heat according to purely physical laws. Probably in the second century B.C., an astounding change took place, whose details remain quite obscure. In addition to the blood, the Chinese came to recognize, at that time, a vaporous agent, qì, to be of vital significance. Qì flowed, most importantly, in the conduits permeating the deeper levels of the limbs and body, and was supplemented or drained not with the pointed blood-letting stone, but with fine needles.

6. The flow of qì pneuma

The character for qì, 氣 (now simplified to 气 in the PRC), is composed of two pictographic components, which combine the meanings of "vapor" (气) and "food" (米). Thus, one could imagine this character as the ideal pictographic representation of a concept that in the Hippocratic writings had a comparable function, namely *physai ek ton perittomaton*, "vapors from food." Conversely, one could also argue that the Hippocratic concept of "vapors from food" is the perfect translation of the original character qì.

Similar to the ancient European concepts of *pneuma* and *spiritus*, qì developed from a limited sense into a complex concept. In medical usage, it fulfilled the concept of a "pneuma," a substance of finest matter that pervades the whole world, as breath flows into the body, but is also bound in food and in drugs, thereby not only linking the body's internal economy with the economy of the macrocosm, but showing them to be one and the same thing. Qì can manifest as anything.

Ancient Chinese medicine associated with qì certain ideas that in many respects appear meaningful even against the background of modern thought. The stomach was considered to be the place from which all organs were supplied with qì extracted from food and drink. Each organ sends its own qì through the blood vessels, so that the state of each of the organs could be felt through the pulse. A dangerous situation arose when the pure qì of only one of the organs could be felt in the beat of the pulse, without any admixture of stomach qì. The prognosis of such a state was highly unfavorable.

Also flowing through the blood vessels and conduits, as well as outside them—the exact morphological identification of these pathways was never settled—were "field camp qì" (营气 *yíng qì*) and "defense qì" (卫气 *wèi qì*), agents whose names were borrowed from the military. It should not surprise anyone how in the late 19th and earlier 20th centuries the ideas of modern medicine, in particular of bacteriology, were adopted in China. In quite different garb, though easily identifiable, notions of defense and immunity appeared in China out of a purely naturalistic context two thousand years ago.

The flow of qì in the body, in the words of the *Inner Canon of the Yellow Thearch*, is "like a circle, without beginning and end." Thus Chinese doctors right from the start took for granted the notion of circulation, even if their notion of circulation differed in detail from the circulation which modern medicine has discovered since Harvey's publications in the 17th century.

One basis of the ancient Chinese concept of circulation—a point brought home by terminology—may have been the significance of irrigation for Chinese agriculture: fields not reached by water dried up. So too it was in the body. Under morbid conditions, whole organ spheres could be deprived of flow, with analogous consequences. The flow moves regularly in one direction, but in pathological states it can change its direction and flow counter to the norm. Of course, blockages are also possible, and lead to morbid accumulations of qì and blood.

7. Sickness and evil

Whether the circulation of qì is disturbed essentially depends on one basic condition: the organism must be vulnerable. The healthy body is capable of defending itself; no evil can enter it from outside. A basic idea that runs through Chinese medicine is that an evil cannot gain access where "right" (正 zhèng) dominates. This maxim, understandable both politically and medically, corresponds to the goal of Confucianism to allow no cause for rebellion and prevent crisis by setting the affairs of state in order early, and leading the people toward correct behavior before things get out of hand.

The political analogy of medicine and statecraft was a natural one for the authors of *The Inner Canon of the Yellow Thearch*; it found expression in the dictum of the classics that the sages intervene therapeutically before a disease has arisen, in the same way as they intervene to impose order before unrest has broken out. The Chinese term for "intervene therapeutically" and "intervene to impose order" is the same (治 zhì).

The medical notion of prevention in the sense of the intervention in the first stages of any change derives from the concern that a focus of rebellion could develop into a widespread conflagration that could threaten the state. This is understandable and also seems plausible from a Western viewpoint. Nevertheless, unlike ancient European medicine, the transfer of political experience to dealing with the body in China excluded the belief in the self-healing capacity of the body. Ancient Chinese medicine almost entirely neglected the *vis medicatrix naturae* (healing power of nature) that European writers again and again affirmed. The allegory of body and state imposed vigilance and a preparedness for immediate intervention at the slightest deviation from a condition believed normal.

The experience of the long period of warring states that preceded the unification of China taught that the organism becomes vulnerable when it shows any weakness, and that this weakness is always a deficiency. Each organ possesses it own qì. This qì is used when an organ is stressed. An abnormal stress causing a deficiency or even an "emptiness" arises for example when the five emotions, each of which is associated with an organ, are unduly stimulated. Excessive grief, for instance, can cause an undue drain on the qì of the lung. This gives rise to a deficiency in the lung, and the empty space can be occupied by cold qì, which penetrates from outside the body when the affected person happens to be exposed to this alien qì. The ancient, very concrete notion of "fullness" in the vessels was given a new interpretation in this context: fullness as the presence of an alien qì in the vessels, the conduits, or organs.

Cold, wind, and heat are natural companions of man, but any one of them becomes an "evil" that creates a morbid "fullness" when it has the opportunity to exploit a deficiency in the body and penetrate where it actually has no business to. Although the principle of the medicine of systematic correspondences is a systematic-functional one, this example nevertheless shows the deep-rootedness of ontic thinking in Chinese medicine as a whole. Illness is always primarily, or at least secondarily, connected with an "evil" located in the wrong place in the body and causing damage. The "evil" can be one of the six climatic influences that gains access to the body and then moves from one functional sphere to another. It can also, in a somewhat abstract sense, be the qì of an organ that is prompted by a deficiency in a neighboring organ to overstep its own borders and occupy the territory of its neighbor. The medical terminology used in traditional Chinese medicine to describe such processes is naturally militaristic in tone.

8. Diagnosis of functional disturbances

When a doctor who felt bound to the tradition of the medicine of systematic correspondence treated a patient, it was necessary for him to determine categorically which evil was afflicting the patient, via what organ the evil (if of exogenous origin) had found its way into the body, where it was currently located in the organism, what damage it had already caused in the economy of qì, and what other spheres it could possibly move into.

It is not known to what extent these theoretical precepts were actually, or could be, applied by Chinese doctors in diagnostic practice. Nevertheless, they laid the foundations for the reputation of the systematic tradition as a holistic medicine. The reputation of holism is justified insofar as this tradition viewed the human organism in diagnosis and therapy as an integrated system of individual parts—in a way very similar to that in which, in the theory of modern medicine, the entirety of physiological processes in the body are understood only against the backcloth of complicated circuits of biochemical and biophysical reactions involving all the organs.

The depot and palace organs, as they are called, formed yīn-yáng pairs closely connecting the internal with the external: the spleen and stomach, the liver and gallbladder, the heart and the small intestine, the lung and the large intestine, the kidney and the urinary bladder, the heart-enclosing network and the triple burner. Each organ was in turn connected with particular processes within the body, with particular emotions, and also with sense organs and their functions. The natural philosophers of ancient China sought to understand and explain relationships between all aspects of the organism with equally complex derivations of the yīn-yáng and five-phase doctrines. For this reason, we speak of "functional spheres," which were assigned to the organs understood as actual morphological entities.

The holism of the systematic-functional tradition of Chinese medicine, which expressed itself in the networking of all components of the individual organism, was complemented by a second holism by which the individual is incorporated into the processes of the universe. In the same way as modern science considers the chemical and physical laws that determine the well-being and suffering of each organism to be operant in the farthest stars, so Chinese observers of nature for two thousand years viewed the relationships between both yīn-yáng and five-phase categories of all being as applicable not only to the individual human being but also to the universe as a whole. In this way, the individual was incorporated into the geographical and climatic conditions of his environment and had to subordinate himself to these conditions in order to stay in health.

The diagnostic structures of the systematic tradition of Chinese medicine underwent an effective elaboration in the first century A.D., the effects of which lasted until the present. Since antiquity, it had been established that the patient had to be examined by four methods, namely inspection, listening and smelling, inquiry, and pulse-taking. Consequently, the best doctor was the one who could see a disease in the patient by mere observation, say, of changes in the complexion. According to the doctrine of the five phases, each organ sphere was externally associated with a particular coloring and a particular area of the face; particular changes in the coloration of the face made it supposedly possible to draw conclusions about morbid changes within the body.

A doctor who did not have the ability to make a diagnosis on the first inspection could draw his conclusions from listening and smelling. Each organ sphere was associated with a particular smell and particular quality of voice; the healer could determine where the evil was located in the body from particular body odors and mouth smells as well as from crying, weeping, or other sounds emitted by the patient.

If this method failed to identify the underlying disease, the doctor could also resort to inquiry. He could ask about the dietary habits, ability to sleep, digestion, pain in the body, and many other factors in order to form a picture of the condition resulting from disease within the body. Only when the hints gleaned by these methods provided no conclusive diagnosis could the doctor then resort to the fourth diagnostic method, pulse-taking.

An early Chinese term for pulse-taking still used today is *kàn mài* (看脉), which literally means "looking at the vessels." This term hails from the time when the condition of the blood vessels and the skin covering them was determined visually. In the century about the beginning of the Christian era, the concept of "vessel" (脉 *mài*) was extended to include the meaning of "movement in the vessels," that is, the beat of the pulse, and from this time the various pulse types were identified as important evidence of the internal state of the body. Pulse diagnosis was the last in the enumeration of the four methods, but for two millennia it has possibly been the most significant.

The *Nàn Jīng* of the 1st century A.D. brought this diagnostic approach to completion, and introduced various methods of pulse diagnosis, which in our Western view are mutually contradictory, but which in traditional Chinese logic are all equally valid since they derive from one and the same basic principle considered valid, namely systematic correspondence.

One method was based on the notion that at the high point of the styloid process below (medial to) the wrist there was an imaginary line, called the "pass" (关 *guān*), as a narrow passage through mountains. When a finger feels the pulse with light pressure above the "pass," i.e., toward the wrist, the pulse offers evidence about the state of the lung and heart. The connection lies in the fact that the imaginary line, the "pass," corresponds to the diaphragm in the human body. The lung and heart are located above this separation, in the yáng area of the body. The lung and the heart therefore manifest in pulse above the "pass" in the yáng region. Below the pass, in the yīn region, the pulse reflects the condition of the liver and kidney, organs which lie below the diaphragm in the yīn region of the body. Right on the pass, the middle of the three fingers feels the state of the spleen, the organ that lies closest to the diaphragm.

A second method of pulse-taking uses the pressure of a single finger. The finger exerts a light pressure in the area of the pass and feels the pulse just below the skin, that is, in a yáng region, which provides information about the lung and heart. Somewhat greater pressure allows the finger to penetrate the level where the pulse of the spleen can be felt. Applying still greater pressure so that the fingertip enters the yīn region and almost reaches the bone, the level of the liver and kidneys is reached.

This method stands alongside yet another by which the finger, by application of different degrees of pressure, feels the state of the five organs each at five distinct levels.

Ancient literature assures that it takes long experience to interpret correctly the information that can be gained from the four diagnostic methods. There are heat conditions that indicate heat in the body, yet there are also heat conditions stemming from underlying cold. There are conditions of the pulse that agree with the other manifestations of illness; there are others that disagree, so that the doctor must possess the knowledge necessary to be able to decide which signs represent the true nature of the patient's disease and what therapy is therefore called for.

9. Qì manipulation therapy

In the systematic-functional view of the illness, no connection between a particular basic disease and its expression is as close as the connection in Western medicine between a number of diseases and their clearly-defined symptoms. Only the latest developments in modern medicine, whereby a variety of particular chemical values of a patient's body are determined in order to make a diagnosis of the underlying disease, have created pictures of basic diseases and their manifestations as diffuse as those the functional tradition of Chinese medicine has dealt with for two thousand years.

A disturbance of qì in the kidney conduit can manifest itself in various ways, and can cause different pathological states. This means that two patients with an identical disturbance of qì in the kidney conduit can nevertheless present different conditions and have to be treated identically irrespective of these apparent differences. Conversely, similar states can develop from different underlying diseases and thus call for different therapy.

The object of treatment is to get to the underlying disease, to the "root" (本 *běn*). The morbid states, called the "tips" of the branches (标 *biāo*), are those things that the doctor sees from outside or that the patient is aware of himself. Treatment can be directed towards the pathological state, but ancient Chinese doctors developed precise standards to determine what states and stages of disease should first be treated by the root or the tips.

It is also possible for two "roots" to coincide in the body when two distinct evils have arisen in or penetrated the body. Of course it takes special skill to trace often disparate pathological states to two diseases existing in parallel. Two conditions, then, are "fought" by different procedures.

Even acupuncture recognized the existence of an ontic evil, which, as an enemy, finds its way into the body and moves about this foreign territory. It differed from the earlier tradition in explaining this evil as qì and in imagining this evil could only penetrate the body when it was given the opportunity to do so. It was no blunder when Chinese writers in later centuries conceived and named therapeutic strategies of acupuncture according to the rules of the art of war.

In this situation, the doctor assumes the role of commander-in-chief: he has to know the territory on which the battle is to take place; he has to try to surround the enemy, to cut his supply lines, and finally to destroy him.

When in the Zhōu period the famous, albeit semi-legendary, wandering healer Biǎn Què (扁鹊) came to audience with the Marquis Huán of Qí, he immediately observed that the marquis was sick and in need of treatment. The marquis responded to this advice saying that he felt quite well. After Biǎn Què had left, the marquis spoke to his entourage, saying that doctors were interested in profit more than anything else and therefore preferred to treat the healthy. Yet Biǎn Què made two further visits and warned with increasing insistence that the marquis should receive treatment, each time without success. At the fourth and last visit, Biǎn Què glimpsed the marquis from a distance and promptly left the court. A messenger sent to ask why he had left so quickly received the following answer from the physician: "when a disease is in the pores of the skin, it can be cured through hot compresses. When it is in the blood vessels, it can be eliminated using pointed stones (i.e., blood-letting). When it advances to the region of the stomach and intestines, it can be treated with medicinal wines. Now that the disease is in the bones, no treatment is of any avail." Five days after the messenger had returned with this answer, the marquis became visibly ill and died.

This anecdote from the historical work the *Shǐ Jì* (史记) from the year 90 B.C. is informative. The ontic understanding of disease is quite patent. The disease represents an independent evil that invades the body as foreign intruders invade a country, and according to the therapeutic imperative of ancient Chinese medicine that complemented the complete prevention of disease, it was to be confronted as early as possible.

The Inner Canon of the Yellow Thearch contains a famous passage that may have already been formulated in the Hàn period (about the beginning of the Christian era):

To follow the laws of yīn and yáng means life; to go against means death. When it is therefore said that the sages of antiquity did not treat those who were already sick, but those who were not sick, and did not intervene where unrest had already broken out, but where there was as yet no unrest, then this is what is meant. When a disease has already broken out, and is only then treated with medicaments, or when unrest has broken out and only then does one intervene to impose order, would that not be just as late as to wait for thirst before digging a well or to wait to go into battle before casting weapons?

Ancient Chinese medical thought is in many respects a political analogy. The concepts of the systematic-functional tradition are identical with the political maxims of Confucianism in many regards. Yet just as it is not possible to prevent every state crisis through good politics, so it is not possible to avoid every illness through appropriate life-style, clothing suited to climatic changes, intake of food adjusted to the seasons, restraint in sexual behavior, a balance of rest and activity, and other aspects of behavior. To lay emphasis on individual behavior nevertheless means to treat before a disease has broken out.

Right at the beginning of the prescription work the *Jīn Guì Yào Luè* (金匮要略), Zhāng Jī, who lived about the year A.D. 200, posed the rhetorical question as to what was actually meant by the statement that the best practitioners of antiquity did not treat those who were already sick, but clearly in a completely different sense. His explanation reads, "When they saw that the liver was diseased, then they knew that the liver was about to transmit [the evil qì] to the spleen. For this reason, they supplemented the spleen [with right qì]. At the end of each season, the spleen flourishes, and cannot contract any evil; at that time, no supplementation should be given. The practitioners of medium ability know nothing of the transmission within the body. When they see a liver disease, they do not solve this problem by supplementing the spleen [with right qì]."

In ancient Chinese medicine, prevention thus poses two approaches: one involving a general avoidance of illness through a *diaita*, as was proposed by ancient European medicine in demands for comprehensive shaping of life-style; another involving the prevention of aggravation, that is, stemming the transmission of evil in the body as early as possible. These thoughts are specifically Chinese since they are closely connected with the doctrine of the five phases and the idea of a conduit system in the body, which were unknown outside China.

Zhāng Jī follows the above-quoted passage with an example of how disease of the liver is to be remedied: The qì of the liver is supplemented with foods or drugs of sour flavor. This is supported with foods and drugs of burning qì and bitter flavor. Drugs with sweet flavor are to be used in order to achieve a regulating balance. Sour flavor penetrates the liver; burning qì and bitter flavor enter the heart; sweet flavor enters the spleen. The spleen is capable of damaging the kidney. When the qì of the kidney is weak, water does not flow. When water does not flow, then the fire qì of the heart blazes and afflicts damage on the lung. When the lung has suffered damage, metal qì cannot move, and when this happens, the qì of the liver increases, and the liver is healed.

Zhāng Jī was the first writer, and for a thousand years to come, the last, to attempt to incorporate the use of drugs into the doctrine of the five phases. The liver is associated with wood, the heart with fire, the spleen with earth, and the kidneys with water. A strengthened spleen means that earth dams the water of the kidney. When water is contained, it fails to subdue fire, which corresponds to the heart. When fire blazes uncontrolled, it melts metal, thereby weakening the lung. Weakened metal is no longer capable of chopping wood, so that the qì of the liver associated with the wood phase can make its recovery.

These thoughts were plausible for Zhāng Jī; for later writers for centuries they were not. The pharmaceutical tradition remained free of the theories of systematic correspondence until the 12th century, developing independently on purely pragmatic and empirical bases. The doctrines of the five phases and of yīn and yáng remained limited to life-style and the tradition of influencing qì. Their only instrument was the needle.

10. Acupuncture

The anecdote about the encounter between the wandering doctor Biǎn Què and Marquis Huán of Qí illustrates nicely the breadth of possibilities for treatment that a doctor had to master if he were to successfully choose appropriate methods for treatment after the beginning stage of illness. The complete spectrum of therapeutic procedures available to Chinese medicine was already set forth in the Mǎwángduī texts of the early 2nd century B.C.: cauterization by burning mugwort at particular points on the skin that were understood to be entry points into the vessels (moxibustion), compresses, fumigations, medicinal baths, petty surgery, magical incantations, magic ritual movements, massage, cupping, and, of course, pharmaceutics. Only acupuncture was missing.

The method of puncturing the skin of a patient with needles to achieve therapeutic effects is first mentioned in the double biography of the ambulant healer Biǎn Què and the grain store administrator Chúnyú Yì (淳于意) in the Shǐ Jì in the year 90 B.C. Biǎn Què used the needle only once to puncture the head of the Crown Prince of the state of Guó (虢) to revive him from a loss of consciousness that had affected him for half a day. The author of the Shǐ Jì did not inform his readers whether Biǎn Què knew of other insertion points and whether he was acquainted with the most fundamental feature of acupuncture, namely the system of conduits, whose qì flow was influenced by needling.

The second half of the double biography offers a clearer hint. Chúnyú Yì (216–ca 150 B.C.) had to defend himself twice, in the years 167 and 154 B.C., against the accusation of medical malpractice. The *Shĭ Jì* records his defense and several evidently exemplary cases of his medical activity. Chúnyú Yì stated that he had been challenged by his teacher to give up treating by drug prescriptions, and to use vessel therapies instead—a clear indication of the antagonism, at least in many circles, between the old tradition of drug therapy and the newly developing qì medicine and acupuncture.

We can infer from the *Shĭ Jì* that Chúnyú Yì followed the instructions of his teacher only in part. He is described as an able physician who found the right treatment for his patients especially through pulse diagnosis and through the use of drugs. To what extent the descriptions of the case histories are authentic can no longer be determined; but they allow the conclusion that around 100 B.C., when Sīmǎ Qiān was writing his work, vessel diagnosis and therapy were already known procedures. Chúnyú Yì, according to the author of the *Shĭ Jì*, felt the pulse and thereby deduced the state of qì in particular organs. This enabled him to determine the cause of the disease (e.g., excessive grief damaging the lung) and the prognosis.

Whether the vessel therapies applied by Chúnyú Yì and other doctors mentioned in the medical case histories included acupuncture or blood-letting in addition to cauterization is not clearly attestable. It is several times stated that he punctured particular vessels, but whether he did this with needles or pointed stones remains unclear. We do know, however, that the terms pointed stone and needle are both mentioned.

The *Shĭ Jì* may have been written precisely at the point in time when needle therapy was replacing blood-letting. Ancient texts convey the impression that puncturing with needles along definite conduit paths was used to drain concrete fullness or supplement deficiencies. *The Inner Canon of the Yellow Thearch* recorded with great anatomical detail the paths of the conduits along which needles were to be inserted.

In 1992, a black-lacquered wooden figure with systematic orange-red linear markings was unearthed in a tomb in Sìchuān dating from the Western Hàn Dynasty (2nd–1st century B.C.). There is every reason to assume that the lines were superficial representations of the conduits within the body, similar to those on the teaching models of the Sòng period over a thousand years later.

Although the pathways of the conduits on the figure do not agree with those traditionally described in texts, this discovery provides some substantiation for the assumption that in the beginning phase of the vessel doctrine, the vessels as such were the sole focus of attention. Only in a second phase did Chinese doctors mark particular points on the skin that they understood as places of entry and exit of qì, which they accordingly called "holes" (穴 xué).

The uncertain dating of the individual historical layers of *The Inner Canon of the Yellow Thearch* poses difficulties for a precise analysis of the development of acupuncture in its early phase. The *Nàn Jīng*, "The Classic of Difficult Issues," from probably the 1st century, may mark a certain conclusion of the early phase. This text concentrated on five, and when the yīn-yáng doctrine was applied, six, insertion openings on the lower leg and forearm, as well as on particular transport openings (俞穴 shū xué) on the chest and back.

Insertion openings on the limbs were named by analogy to the course of Chinese rivers. The first hole was the source (井 jǐng), followed by the brook (荥 yíng), the place where the rivers became navigable (俞 shū), the stream (经 jīng), and finally by the confluence (合 hé). The sixth insertion point lay between the point where the rivers become navigable and the stream point, and was given the topographically meaningful designation of "plain" (原 yuán).

Ancient Chinese sources indicate that it was a mistake to treat manifest forms of disease with needles. Needles were considered to provide a subtle stimulus capable of remedying disturbances in their early stages. This reservation was not held to. According to writers over the following centuries up to the dissolution of this tradition in the 19th century, acupuncture could cure many different diseases, a claim illustrated by a wealth of literature. One of the most comprehensive prescription works, the *Pǔ Jì Fāng* (普济方, "Prescriptions for Comprehensive Aid") from the early 15th century, for example, enumerates no fewer than 290 conditions for which acupuncture was thought to be effective.

A detailed analysis of the development of acupuncture over this period is not available. Our present state of knowledge nevertheless allows the assertion that treatment with needles remained the focal therapeutic means of the medicine of systematic correspondences until the 12th century. Only then was the time ripe for the theories of systematic correspondence, i.e., the doctrines of yīn and yáng and the five phases, to be extended to the effects of drugs in the organism. Acupuncture gradually freed itself from the limited notions of real fullness or emptiness in the vessels. It came to consider in addition emptiness in the abstract sense as lack of right qì, and fullness as the presence of unright qì in the organs and their functional spheres. Furthermore, it served to treat stagnation and counterflow in the flow of qì through the vessels.

Doctors thought up numerous techniques in order to improve the effect of needles, e.g., by heating them, by inserting them obliquely in or against the direction of qì flow (to achieve a supplementing or draining effect respectively), and by inserting needles as the patient breathed in or out.

With the exception of the prescription works of Zhāng Jī around A.D. 200, two distinct traditions of medical literature developed after the Hàn Dynasty: pharmaceutical and prescription literature that did without the theories of yīn and yáng and the five phases, and hardly cared about the state of qì, and acupuncture literature that cultivated precisely these notions. To what extent the two traditions were strictly separate is uncertain. Sūn Sīmiǎo (孙思邈 581–682?), the most famous physician of the Táng period, who has been revered since the 13th century as the god of pharmacy, was versed in acupuncture as well as pharmacy.

CHAPTER THREE
THE DOCTRINE OF THE FIVE PERIODS AND SIX QÌ

1. The regularity of climatic phenomena

The centuries after the conclusion of the formative phase of Chinese medicine toward the end of the Hàn Dynasty are not characterized by any conspicuous dynamic of medical knowledge. Zhāng Jī (张机, around A.D. 200) was the last innovator, yet his contribution to the unification of the pharmaceutical tradition with the theoretical tradition was not accepted. Huángfǔ Mì (皇甫谧, 214–282) was intensively engaged in acupuncture, however his *Zhēn Jiǔ Jiǎ Yǐ Jīng* (针灸甲乙经), "Canon of Acupuncture and Moxibustion," offered no basic progress. Sūn Sīmiǎo (孙思邈, 581–682?) compiled voluminous prescription works, but he provided no impetus to thought.

Against this background, the doctrine of the five periods and six qì (五运六气 *wǔ yùn liù qì*) is of particular interest. The highly complex conceptual structure suddenly appeared without any indication of a development phase in the revision by Wáng Bīng (王冰) of *Elementary Questions* (素问 *sù wèn*) of *The Inner Canon of the Yellow Thearch* at the beginning of the 7th century. Wáng Bīng indicated in his preface that he had added this new element to the text—a third of the complete text of *Elementary Questions* that has been handed down to the present—though he did not name any sources. To this day, we know of no text from the time before Wáng Bīng's revision of *Elementary Questions* that contains comparable ideas. The analysis of the seven "Comprehensive Discourses" (大论 *dà lùn*), as the corresponding treatises in *The Inner Canon of the Yellow Thearch* are referred to, shows very clearly that here different traditions converged, so that some prior development of these ideas must be presumed.

The doctrine of the five periods and six qì serves to explain relationships that the ancient Chinese observers of nature were convinced of perceiving between climatic changes on the one hand and the development of a wide spectrum of natural phenomena including human health and disease on the other. Clearly, the concepts of the five periods and six qì were introduced in order to distinguish and characterize climatic features of well-defined time spans. Taking recourse to notions of a cyclical recurrence of calendar dates and with the support of the yīn-yáng and five-phase doctrine, the creators of the doctrine of the five phases and six qì sought to impose order on what at first sight appeared to have no order, i.e., the occurrence of rain, wind, dryness, cold, and heat in the course of the four seasons and over the years.

The knowledge of definite laws governing climatic change enabled man, as the creators of this doctrine believed, not only to gain an understanding of production, growth, maturation, and death of numerous natural phenomena in general, but also allowed man, above all, to integrate himself into the eternal laws by which his existence was fulfilled. In the same way, the individual could secure survival and well-being through subordination to the laws enacted by a ruler in the state, so man could secure life and avoid early death through obedience to the laws formulated by an unseen natural power. And just as to go against the laws of society ends in punishment, those who go against the laws of nature perish. It is therefore not surprising that the doctrine of the five periods and six qì borrows its terminology for certain focal concepts from social life, and in many of its statements reads like a political metaphor. The 68th treatise of *Elementary Questions*, for instance, is a clear example of the conservative attitude of Chinese medicine in general and of the doctrine of the five periods and six qì in particular. It states that opposition is the basis of change, and change is the basis of disease.

In order to describe and analyze long-term cycles of recurring climatic phenomena, ancient Chinese observers of nature combined two series of symbols, which for many centuries had been used to calculate periods of the calendar, namely the ten heavenly stems (天干 *tiān gān*) and the twelve earthly branches (地支 *dì zhī*), with the doctrines of yīn and yáng and five phases. The combination of the five phases with the ten heavenly stems led to a sequence of five periodically recurring periods of a given characteristic, the so-called five periods (五运 *wǔ yùn*). The combination of the yīn-yáng doctrine extended to three yīn and three yáng categories of all being with the twelve earthly branches led to the sequence of six (climatic) qì. As each year is associated with a particular combination of a heavenly stem and earthly branch, each year appeared linked in a specific way to climatic features, which in turn were related to the six qì and five phases.

The doctrine of the five periods and six qì is based on the assumption that even apparently unusual climatic events form part of a regular recurrence of particular constellations ensuing from the combination of specific qualities of periods and qì resulting in excessive dominances or weaknesses of these qualities. Knowledge of these constellations and their regularity allows abnormal climatic conditions to be predicted so that people can safeguard their health by preparing themselves through appropriate adjustment of behavior.

2. Calculation of constellations

The first step towards this goal consists in the choice of a method that makes it possible to calculate the constellations within each year and over periods of years, and to derive from these calculations the characteristic features of these constellations.

In ancient China, the so-called heavenly stems and earthly branches were used to denote the days and years. The ten heavenly stems are as follows:

jiǎ 甲 , *yǐ* 已 , *bǐng* 丙 , *dīng* 丁 , *wù* 戊 ,
jǐ 己 , *gēng* 庚 , *xīn* 辛 , *rén* 壬 , *guǐ* 癸 .

This sequence as a whole possesses a yáng quality.

The twelve earthly stems are as follows:

zǐ 子 , *chǒu* 丑 , *yín* 寅 , *mǎo* 卯 , *chén* 辰 , *sì* 巳 ,
wǔ 午 , *wèi* 未 , *shēn* 申 , *yǒu* 酉 , *xū* 戊 , *hài* 亥 .

This sequence as a whole possesses a yīn quality.

A combination of a stem and a branch (e.g., *jiǎ-zǐ*, *jiǎ-chǒu*, *yǐ-zǐ*, *yǐ-chǒu*, etc.) results in a total of 60 possible pairings. These pairings may be used to denote a series of sixty years, and to characterize each year with specific climatic features.

Each year in a cycle of 60 years thus has its own label using a combination of a heavenly stem and earthly branch. The heavenly stem characterizes the period of the year; the earthly stem denotes the qì of the year.

Each cycle of 60 years begins with the combination of the stem *jiǎ* and the earthly branch *zǐ*; the first year is thus a *jiǎ-zǐ* year. The second year in each cycle is a *yǐ-chǒu* year, the third a *bǐng-yín* year, the fourth a *dīng-mǎo* year, and so forth up to the tenth, the *guǐ-yǒu* year. The eleventh to 20th years are called *jiǎ-xū*, *yǐ-hài*, *bǐng-zǐ* up to *guǐ-wèi*, etc.

The enumeration of the years in the dual sequence of stems and branches is not just a serial arrangement. The stems and branches have very specific qualitative meanings, as can be seen in two respects. First, they are classified as yīn and yáng respectively. Here, stems and branches with uneven numbers are yáng and those with even numbers are yīn (see Tables 1 and 2), and yáng stems can only be combined with yáng branches and yīn stems only with yīn branches. Second, the stem and branch combinations of each year represent correspondences of different yīn-yáng categories to the five phases.

This means that as soon as the stem and branch designations of a particular year are known, its climatic features can be calculated on the basis of the associations of each stem and branch within the five periods and six qì.

1	2	3	4	5	6	7	8	9	10
甲	已	丙	丁	戊	己	庚	辛	壬	癸
jiǎ	yǐ	bǐng	dīng	wù	jǐ	gēng	xīn	rén	guǐ
yáng	yīn	yáng	yīn	yáng	yīn	yáng	yīn	yáng	yīn

Table 1. The yīn-yáng associations of heavenly stems.

1	2	3	4	5	6	7	8	9	10	11	12
子	丑	寅	卯	辰	巳	午	未	申	酉	戌	亥
zǐ	chǒu	yín	mǎo	chén	sì	wǔ	wèi	shēn	yǒu	xū	hài
yáng	yīn	yáng	yīn	yáng	yīn	yáng	yīn	yáng	yīn	yáng	yīn

Table 2. The yīn-yáng associations of the earthly branches.

3. The five periods

"Five periods" is a generic term for the quality of periodically recurring phenomena, including qì, that are associated with the five phases metal, wood, water, fire, and earth and that characterize either five consecutive years or five seasons within a year. A "period" can thus refer both to a whole year as well as one of the five seasons.

The concept of the five periods is closely associated with the concept of the five phases in the doctrine of the five phases.

Thus, the relationships of domination and revenge, and of engendering and overcoming between the individual periods, are identical with those between the individual phases. Yet there are differences, as the following table shows.

jiă	*yĭ*	*bĭng*	*dīng*	*wù*	*jĭ*	*gēng*	*xīn*	*rén*	*guĭ*
甲	已	丙	丁	戊	己	庚	辛	壬	癸
yáng	*yīn*	*yáng*	*yīn*	*yáng*	*yīn*	*yáng*	*yīn*	*yáng*	*yīn*
wood		fire		earth		metal		water	
east		south		center		west		north	

Table 3. The association of heavenly stems with the five phases.

jiă	*yĭ*	*bĭng*	*dīng*	*wù*	*jĭ*	*gēng*	*xīn*	*rén*	*guĭ*
甲	已	丙	丁	戊	己	庚	辛	壬	癸
earth	metal	water	wood	fire	earth	metal	water	wood	fire

Table 4. The association of heavenly stems with the periods (linear).

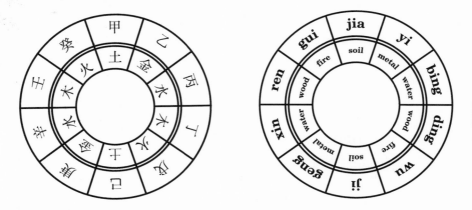

Diagram 1. The association of heavenly stems
with the periods (cyclical).

From Table 4, we can see that the ten stems are twice divided among the five periods, with the latter arranged according to the sequence of engendering. In a cyclical representation, each period is associated with two heavenly stems opposite each other, one of which is yáng and the other of which is yīn.

The annual periods are usually referred to by the names of the five phases. Alternatively, they are known by the names of the five musical notes. Parallel to the association of the voice with the periods, one note is ascribed to two stems. These are differentiated not according to yīn or yáng, but according to "major" and "minor," although the sense is the same. The note gōng, for example, stands for the period Earth.

In the doctrine of the five periods and six qì, earth is associated with the stems jiǎ and jǐ. Jiǎ is a yáng stem, and hence the note gōng is a "major gōng" note when it stands for the yáng stem jiǎ. Jǐ is yīn stem, hence the note gōng is a "minor gōng" note when it stands for a yīn stem jǐ. The complete schema is set forth in the following table:

gōng 宮	earth	jiǎ gōng	major gōng	yáng gōng
		jǐ gōng	minor gōng	yīn gōng
shāng 商	metal	gēng shāng	major shāng	yáng shāng
		guǐ shāng	minor shāng	yīn shāng
jué 角	wood	rén jué	major jué	yáng jué
		dīng jué	minor jué	yīn jué
zhǐ 徵	fire	wù zhǐ	major zhǐ	yáng zhǐ
		guǐ zhǐ	minor zhǐ	yīn zhǐ
yǔ 羽	water	bǐng yǔ	major yǔ	yáng yǔ
		xīn yǔ	minor yǔ	yīn yǔ

Table 5. The five notes which stand for annual periods.

The period associated with a year is an important indication for the climatic situation to be expected in this year. It was therefore also called a "central period" (中运 zhōng yùn) since it runs the whole year, irrespective of which of the six qì were active above, i.e., in the first half of the year, or below, i.e., in the latter half of the year.

Because the qì that proceeds with the annual, or central, period exerts so dominant an influence on the climate of the whole year, it was also called an "annual period" (岁运 *suì yùn*) or "great period" (大运 *dà yùn*).

The annual period can be "excessive" or "inadequate." All annual periods that are associated with yáng stems (namely *jiǎ*, *bǐng*, *wù*, *gēng*, and *rén*) are by definition "excessive"; all annual periods associated with yīn stems (namely *yǐ*, *dīng*, *jǐ*, *xīn*, and *guǐ*) are "inadequate." Although this might give the impression that the climate of the year must be either "excessive" or "inadequate," there are constellations that lead to a balanced qì.

4. The three arrangements

Years with a different annual period are characterized by different climatic conditions. In the doctrine of the five periods and six qì, weakness and fullness, increase and decrease serve to express notions of excessive, inadequate, and balanced. These three states are called the "three arrangements" (三记 *sān jì*). Since each of the five periods can appear in specific constellations in one of these three arrangements, a total of 15 arrangements are possible, of which each has a particular name:

A year with the balanced qì

> Wood period: Widespread Harmony
>
> Fire period: Ascending Brilliance
>
> Earth period: Complete Transformation
>
> Metal period: Secured Balance
>
> Water period: Quiet Adaptation

In a year with inadequate qì

> Wood period: Endangered Harmony
>
> Fire period: Suppressed Light

Earth period: Inferior Supervision

Metal period: Accepted Change

Water period: Dried-Up River

In a year with excessive qì

Wood period: Effusive Growth

Fire period: Bright Daylight

Earth period: Prominent Mound

Metal period: Solid Formation

Water period: Overflowing River

Each of these names refers to particular developments affecting animals, fruits, grains, flavors, the organs and functional spheres of the body, diseases, the climate, and many other things in the year in question.

"Excessive" means that in a given year the qì that proceeds with the annual period exerts particularly violent influences on the climate. When, for example, the annual period is "excessive" in a year associated with the annual period Earth, then the whole climate of this year is characterized by rain and dampness. Diseases in such a year are primarily those that are connected with dampness of the spleen and stomach (and hence digestion) since these functional spheres are related to earth in the doctrine of the five phases.

Conversely, when the annual period is inadequate in a year associated with the annual period belonging to earth, then the influence of the qì of water and dampness is reduced in the overall climatic situation of the year. Because the qì of earth is inadequately developed, the qì of wood, which in the doctrine of the five phases is capable of overcoming earth, takes advantage of the weakness of earth and imposes its influence. In such a year, the characteristics of a year of the wood period make themselves felt, i.e., excessive wind is to be expected since wind is the climatic manifestation of the wood period. Such a constellation also has an unfavorable effect on the spleen and stomach, that is, the functional sphere of digestion, since the weakness of earth qì renders both organs associated with earth susceptible to damage by wind evil.

In concrete, increased lack of appetite, sensation of fullness, rumbling intestines and diarrhea, and increased mental unrest and depression are to be expected. In extreme cases, people are confused and easily irritated; dizziness and headache are common. Those who in such situations experience pain in the sides and suffer from violent vomiting, and in whom movement in the vessels is no longer to be felt at a very specific acupuncture point are bound to die.

The seven "Comprehensive Discourses" from the seventh century in *The Inner Canon of the Yellow Thearch* and many works of the following centuries contained detailed enumerations of the consequences of each possible individual constellation on the "myriad creatures."

5. Host periods, visitor periods, and the five steps

The metaphorical designation of the host periods (主运 *zhǔ yùn*) and visitor periods (客运 *kè yùn*) rests on the notion that the host is the regular and lasting occupant of a property, whereas visitors come and go at irregular intervals, and are not necessarily expected. In the doctrine of the five periods and six qì, each year is divided into a series of "five steps" (五步 *wǔ bù*) each of equal length. The host is responsible for the regular climatic situation of the step he watches over. The sequence of hosts that are responsible for the climate of the individual steps over the duration of years is identical for each year. The first host in the year is always the wood period, the second is the fire period, the third is the earth period, the fourth is the metal period, and the fifth is the water period.

The hosts (and also the visitors), though, do not bear the names of the five phases, but also—as occasionally the annual periods do—the designations of the five notes. Thus the first period is called *jué*, the second *zhǐ*, the third *gōng*, the fourth *shāng*, and the fifth *yǔ*.

Each step in the course of a year is associated not only with the host, but also with a visitor. The visitors are responsible for abnormal changes in the climate of the five seasons. In contrast to the fixed sequence of the hosts, that of the visitors varies from year to year.

The first visitor period, that is, the visitor period associated with the first of the five steps, is always identical with the annual period. In the first year of a 60-year cycle, for example, a *jiǎ-zǐ* year, the annual period is yáng and earth, because the heavenly stem of this year, *jiǎ*, is yáng. In such a year, the visitor is also yáng and earth. A yáng earth visitor bears the designation "major *gōng*." The remaining four visitors of this year follow the order of the sequence of engendering of the five phases: wood is followed by fire, then by earth, metal, and water.

6. The six qì

The six qì are the conceptual opposite of the five periods. Just as the five periods appear on three conceptual levels (annual period, host period, and visitor period), so the six qì also appear on three levels, namely "qì controlling heaven," "host qì," and "visitor qì." The concept of "qì controlling heaven" (司天之气 *sī tiān zhī qì*) is somewhat more complex than the concept of the annual period; it stands for a climatic influence over a whole year, over the first half of the year and over the third visitor qì.

In general Chinese medical usage, the term "six qì" refers to cold, summerheat, dryness, dampness, wind, and fire as external qì that can penetrate the body to give rise to illness. There is no relationship between the sequence of the causes of disease and the climatic changes over the course of a year. In the doctrine of the five periods and six qì, by contrast, the term "six qì" refers to the changing climatic conditions within the space of a year. Their names are as follows:

Major yáng, namely cold and water

Yáng brilliance, dryness and metal

Minor yáng, fire

Major yīn, dampness and earth

Minor yīn, heat

Ceasing yīn, wind and wood

The three yīn and three yáng categorizations of the six qì are understood as direct quantitative hints. They express a sequence of gradual increase and decrease in the yīn and yáng qualities of the six qì in the cyclical order of the latter. Strikingly, the strongest yáng category, major yáng, is associated with cold, whereas the weakest yáng category, minor yáng, is associated with fire. No explanation for the unusual categorization exists. The association of minor yáng with fire and minor yīn with heat are reversed in many associational contexts.

Close relationships exist between the six qì and the five phases. Ceasing yīn qì, which is associated with wind and wood, corresponds to wood in the five phases. Major yīn qì, which is associated with dampness, corresponds to earth, which is also associated with dampness, etc. An obvious obstacle for a close parallel is that the six qì are numerically dissonant with the five phases. In the doctrine of the five periods and six qì, the resulting discrepancy is solved or evaded in either of two ways. One procedure is to leave out one qì (namely fire) completely; the other is to divide one of the phases (namely fire) into two (fire and ministerial fire). From the late Sòng, the designations "ruler fire" and "ministerial fire" became current.

7. The six steps of the host qì and visitor qì

Regular climatic changes, which occur in the course of a six-step division of a year, are assigned to the six host qì. This means that each host qì is associated with one of the six steps. The order of the six host qì is identical for each year; it begins with the qì of the wood, and corresponds to the relationships of engendering in the five phases.

First qì: ceasing yīn, wind and wood

Second qì: minor yīn, ruler fire

Third qì: minor yáng, ministerial fire

Fourth qì: major yīn, dampness and earth

Fifth qì: yáng brilliance, dryness and metal

Sixth qì: major yáng, cold and water

The climatic conditions the host qì stand for thus coincide with the regular climatic changes over the course of the four seasons, spring, summer, autumn, and winter. The "Comprehensive Discourses" in *The Inner Canon of the Yellow Thearch* make it clear that, in contrast to the usual Chinese calendar, the exact number of revolutions of the sun was made the basis for calculating the six steps in the course of the year. Each step was given a length of 60.875 days. Over a whole year, this means a length of 365.25 days, so that every fourth year an intercalary day has to be added. Ancient Chinese astronomers thus came very close to the modern calculation of 365.2422 days for each solar year. A period of four years was given the designation "arrangement." A cycle of twelve years, corresponding to a cycle of twelve earthly branches, thus comprises three "arrangements":

zǐ, chǒu, yín, mǎo: 1st arrangement

chén, sì, wǔ, wèi: 2nd arrangement

shēn, yǒu, xū, hài: 3rd arrangement

The six visitor qì, too, each extend their influence over one of a total of six steps of equal duration. The cyclical order of these steps is nevertheless not identical with those of the steps of the host qì. They follow the quantitative sequence of the three yīn and three yáng qì:

First yīn: ceasing yīn, wind and wood

Second yīn: minor yīn, ruler fire

Third yīn: major yīn, dampness and earth

First yáng: minor yáng, ministerial fire

Second yáng: yáng brilliance, dryness and metal

Third yáng: major yáng, cold and water

Like the five-visitor period, the first visitor qì varies from year to year. It depends on the earthly branch associated with each year. As soon as the earthly branch of a particular year is known, it is possible to determine the qì controlling heaven of this year, and from this work out the order of the six-visitor qì of the year in question. To this end, it is important to know the relationships between the yearly earthly branches and the six yīn and yáng qì.

8. The association of the twelve earthly branches with qì

In the doctrine of the five periods and six qì, the correspondences between the twelve earthly branches and the qì— as the correspondences between the ten heavenly stems and the periods—follow their own rules. In order to establish the connections between the ten heavenly stems and the twelve earthly branches on the one hand and the periods and qì on the other, the normal five-phase relationships have to be disregarded.

In the doctrine of the five phases, the following associations between the twelve earthly branches, the six qì, and the four seasons apply:

yín	*mǎo*	*chén*	*sì*	*wǔ*	*wèi*	*shēn*	*yǒu*	*xū*	*hài*	*zǐ*	*chǒu*
寅	卯	辰	巳	午	未	申	酉	戌	亥	子	丑
wood	soil		fire	soil		metal		soil	water		soil

Table 6. The association of the earthly branches with the five phases (linear)

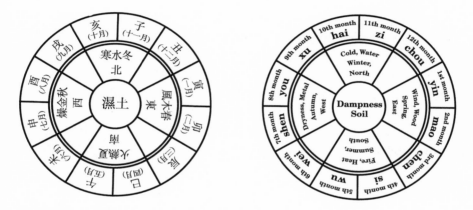

Diagram 2. The association of the earthly branches with the five phases and the twelve months (cyclical).

We can see from Diagram 2 that the twelve earthly branches, starting from the 11th month of the previous year, are each assigned to one of the twelve months of the year. This means that the twelve earthly branches do not coincide exactly with the twelve months of one year. According to the doctrine of the five phases, earth is active in the third and last month of each of the four seasons. Therefore, the third, sixth, ninth, and twelfth month are associated with major yīn, i.e., with dampness and earth. The remaining eight months are ascribed to the remaining four of the five phases.

In the doctrine of the five periods and six qì, in contrast to the doctrine of the five phases, the relationships between the six qì and the twelve earthly stems manifest in association with years, not with months. Here the following relationships apply:

zǐ	chǒu	yín	mǎo	chén	sì
wǔ	wèi	shēn	yǒu	xū	hài
minor yín	major yín	minor yáng	yáng brilliance	major yáng	ceasing yín
ruling fire	earth	ministerial fire	metal	water	wood
--	dampness	--	dryness	cold	wind

Table 7. The association of the earthly branches with the qì (linear).

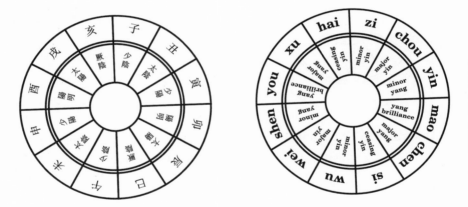

Diagram 3. The association of the earthly branches with the qì (cyclical).

In the correspondences between the ten stems and the periods, the sequence of the ten stems is divided into two sequences from one to five and six to ten, each of which is associated with the five periods (see Diagram 1 above).

The correspondence between the twelve earthly branches and the qì follows the same pattern. The twelve branches are divided into two sequences from one to six and from seven to twelve. Each of the two sequences is connected with the six qì. In a circular representation, we consequently find a pattern in which both earthly branches, which are ascribed to the same qì, in each case appear opposite each other.

On the basis of these diagrams it is now very easy to calculate the qì controlling heaven that are to be expected in a given year.

9. The qì controlling heaven and the qì at the fountain

While the host and visitor periods and the host and visitor qì determine the climatic characteristics of the five or six steps in the course of a year, the qì controlling heaven, also called heavenly qì, like the annual period, is responsible for the influence over a whole year. The qì controlling heaven of a year is the qì associated with the earthly branch of the year. In *jiǎ-zǐ* years, for example, the earthly branch *zǐ* and the qì controlling heaven are minor yīn qì, i.e., ruler fire. Within a 60-year cycle, ten years have the earthly branch *zǐ* or *wǔ*. In these ten years, qì controlling heaven is thus always minor yīn qì, i.e., ruler fire. In all these years, ruler fire qì thus exerts a determining influence. In the terminology of the doctrine of the five periods and six qì, this influence, however, is designated with a political metaphor; texts speak, for example, of the "policy of major yáng qì" and the "policy of yáng brilliance qì," etc.

Besides the division of each year into the five steps of the periods and the six steps of the qì, a division of the year into two halves is also significant for working out the basic climatic features and hence for determining what influences on the health and sickness of the organism are to be expected. The qì that watches over the first half of the year likewise bears the designation "qì controlling heaven," which stands in opposition to the qì of the second half of the year, the "qì at the fountain" (在泉 之气 *zài quán zhī qì*). The names of these qì can be traced back to the ancient notion of nine heavens in the firmament, and nine fountains in the earth, so that "qì at the fountain" is ultimately nothing more than another name for the qì of the earth.

Finally, calculation of the visitor qì in the course of the year shows that the climatic situation during the presence of the third visitor qì coincides with climatic influences exerted by qì controlling heaven. Parallel to this, the climate during the sixth step corresponds to the influences of qì at the fountain.

The ascription of the qì controlling heaven to the third qì and qì at the fountain to the sixth qì gives rise to a further designation for the remaining four steps in the course of the year, as is shown in the following diagram.

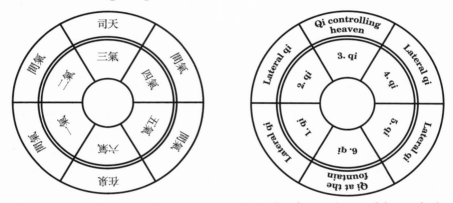

Diagram 4. Qì controlling heaven, qì at the fountain, and lateral qì.

Accordingly, the second qì is understood as right lateral qì and the fourth qì as left lateral qì of qì controlling heaven; the first qì is viewed as left lateral qì and the fifth qì as right lateral qì of qì at the fountain.

In relevant Chinese medical texts, the combined effects of qì controlling heaven, qì at the fountain, and lateral qì, all of which together constitute the visitor qì, on the climate, and hence on the birth and growth of plants and animals, as well as on the genesis and development of diseases in the human organism, are accorded a special significance. In this regard, the influence of qì controlling heaven would appear to exceed the influence of the annual period. The question therefore arose, why was it possible for the organism to be afflicted with sickness even in years in which, according to all calculations, the qì of the annual period was balanced. The answer given in the seven "Comprehensive Discourses" in *The Inner Canon of the Yellow Thearch* is that qì controlling heaven controls the annual period.

The unknown author enumerates the many consequences, say, of minor yáng qì as qì controlling heaven: in the first half of the year, an extremely hot summer, cough, colds, nosebleeds, blocked or runny nose, mouth sores, and alternating cold and heat, and swelling. In the second half of the year, heart pain and stomach ache. An important detail that comes out in the texts is that one and the same qì can cause very different effects depending on whether it is active in the first or second half of the year.

10. Domination, revenge, and resistance

In order to determine the climatic conditions at a particular point in time in the course of a year or for the year as a whole, numerous coordinates from annual periods, host periods, and visitor periods, as well as the host qì, qì controlling heaven, and lateral qì have to be taken into consideration, each against the background of its yīn-yáng and five-phase categorizations and of its own sequences. Yet this is insufficient in itself. In the succession of climatic qì and hence their influence on the processes of becoming, flourishing, illness, and death of all living beings, including man, further relationships between the possible phases are to be taken into account. These relationships are primarily the sequences of domination and revenge as well as domination and resistance. The terminological designations of these relationships are rooted in clear sociopolitical analogies and hence were self-evident to a broad population.

The basic idea of the succession of domination and revenge rests on the notion that an extreme climatic influence on health, when its normal period of dominance comes to an end, is followed by an opposing climatic influence of equally extreme intensity. Such a succession is only possible in years with an inadequate annual period. In such a case, a period that, according to the overcoming relationships of the five periods, is capable of over-coming takes advantage of the weakness of the annual period and exerts its influence. After a certain time, the period that is normally engendered by the weak period (in this case the annual period) comes to take its revenge on the dominant period (which took advantage of the weakness of the mother period) for the humiliation caused to the mother.

In concrete, this means that when the annual period is associated with wood, the metal period takes advantage of the weakness of the annual period, and dominates during the latter's domination period. As a result, there is extreme dryness and cold. The fire period finally comes and takes revenge for the mother. Extreme heat follows the extreme dryness. In this situation, the minor yáng qì dominates and produces feelings of fear, spasm, cough, nosebleed, vexation, twitching of the eyes, mouth sores, vomiting, dry throat, and great thirst. Noteworthy here is the fact that diseases that a minor yáng qì provokes when it takes revenge for the humiliation of the mother period are not identical in every respect with those it causes when it takes advantage of a weakness of another period itself, thereby, as it were, dominating illegitimately. In any event, of course, the lung is the damaged organ, since fire has ascendancy over metal, and the lung is the organ of the metal period.

The six qì can also confront each other in domination and revenge, but here the succession obeys different rules than between the periods. As in real life, domination provokes revenge among the various qì, and the resulting domination triggers new revenge, and so forth. This goes on until the parties in question gradually become exhausted and finally return to normality.

It is interesting to note that a visitor qì is understood to be incapable of avenging the excesses of a host qì. Moreover, the notion developed that there are also situations in which a domination is not avenged by the son of the dominated mother, but that the dominated qì itself—in the sense of pressure producing counterpressure—musters strength to offer resistance.

Numerous other rules lead to an extremely complicated calculation of climatic influences on human health. Many years are characterized by particular constellations and are given designations that reflect the characteristics. For example, a year in which the annual period and the qì controlling heaven have the same phase association is called "Heavenly Talisman." A year in which the phase association of the annual period and annual branch are the same is called "Year Convergence." A year in which the annual period and qì at the fountain have the same phase association, and in which the annual stem and annual branch are yáng is called "Identical with a Heavenly Talisman."

If it is established that there is a dangerous qì dominating at a particular time, then the harm to be expected is avoided primarily by means of medicinal measures. The basic principle of therapy for the dominance of a particular qì is to take drugs of opposite flavor and to eliminate those qì from the body that could be strengthened by the dominant qì. Adjustment of lifestyle with regard to eating and drinking, sleeping and waking, sexual behavior, and clothing further contribute to maintaining health.

CHAPTER FOUR
OPHTHALMOLOGY

1. Eye diseases in earlier literature

Very early on, Chinese writers began to devote separate writings to the basic facets that comprise Chinese medicine, as indeed any medical system. The oldest of such known special texts from the centuries before and after the beginning of the Christian era directed attention to theory, to pharmaceutical prescriptions, to individual descriptions of pharmaceutical drugs, to other forms of therapy (especially acupuncture and moxibustion), and to diagnosis. At least since the Táng period, numerous works have appeared on the subject of specific areas of medicine in the sense of modern specialties. The most noteworthy of these are gynecology, pediatrics, and ophthalmology. Here, we discuss the last of these.

The oracle inscriptions of the late Shāng of about 1000 B.C. contained references to eye diseases. Literature of the Zhōu and the early Hàn period variously describes blindness and simple massage methods to strengthen the eyes. The "Classic of the Mountains and Seas" (山海经 *shān hǎi jīng*, 8th–1st century B.C.) named substances that prevent blindness by means of magical correspondences. The *Huái Nán Zǐ* (淮南子) from the 2nd century B.C. described a plant drug to this day used to relieve inflammation of the eye as suitable "for treatment of the eyes."

The Mǎwángduī texts recommend treatment by cauterization for various kinds of pain in the eyes and canthi; the moxa cones were not to be applied to the eyes themselves, but to particular conduits, whose pathways connected with the various possible locations of pain.

The "Scripture on the Vessels" (脉书 *mài shū*), a text from the 2nd century B.C., which was unearthed from Zhāngjiāshān, describes connections to the conduits in clear detail. It states, for example, that the so-called ear conduit was responsible for "pain in the outer canthi," "pain in the cheeks," and "deafness."

Thus, the basis had been laid for a notion that characterizes traditional Chinese ophthalmology to this day. A large proportion of eye diseases are transmitted from particular organs via the conduit system. When these organs contract an evil that is then transmitted through the conduit to the eyes, the result is a pathological condition whose cause is the disease of an organ.

Xún Zǐ (荀子), the philosopher of the 3rd century B.C., was one of the first to describe the relationship between the heart—not as a concrete organ, but as the seat of knowledge and the emotions—and the eyes. External stimuli that damage the heart as well as the eyes result not only from lasciviousness, and in particular debauchery, but also from "bad music."

The Guǎn Zǐ (管子), a work allegedly from the 3rd or 2nd century B.C., shows for the first time the close connection between the eyes and state of the liver, thereby introducing the most important etiological, diagnostic, and therapeutic concept in Chinese ophthalmology.

2. Morphological details and eye surgery

The Inner Canon of the Yellow Thearch, whose extant contents were written between the 2nd century B.C. and the 8th century A.D., differentiated several morphological regions of the eye, and mentions ailments of the eye such as blindness, exophthalmus, swellings under the eyes, yellowing, pain and reddening, tumorous lesions of the canthus, photophobia, and strabismus. The eye could be affected by these pathologies as an autonomous organ when a cause of disease acted directly on the eye. As a rule, however, *The Inner Canon of the Yellow Thearch* interprets the eye as being an integral part of the internal organism.

Problems in the body's interior do not necessarily, but may, manifest in problems of the eye. The pupil reflects the state of the bones. The "dark" part of the eye reflects the sinews, the "white" part of the eye reflects qì, the eyelids reflect the flesh, etc. In accordance with the doctrine of systematic correspondence, the eyes take on a red coloring when the heart is affected, a white coloring when the lung is affected, a black coloring when the kidney is affected, a yellow coloring when the spleen is affected, and a green coloring when the liver is affected.

The Inner Canon of the Yellow Thearch mentions a morphological connection between the eye and the brain, by which, for example, an evil from the back of the head may penetrate the eye via the brain. When the evil reaches the brain, the brain can turn, so that the eye-brain connection becomes tensed. As a consequence, the patient has the feeling that everything is turning around him. When the evil finally reaches the eyes, then the eyes lose their coordination and the patient sees everything double. When supply of qì through the eye-brain connection to the eye is interrupted the patient dies within 36 hours.

This example shows clearly the status attributed to morphological realities at the beginning of the development of Chinese medicine. It is not known from what sources—possibly outside China—knowledge of a bridge between the eye and the brain came; characteristically, and unlike Aristotle and numerous other investigators in Europe, no one in China showed any interest in dissecting the eye to investigate the physical nature of the organ of vision. When in the Táng and in subsequent centuries questions about the nature of the eyeball were discussed as a result of Indian promptings, Chinese writers quoted Indian texts or raised considerations of their own, but never did such questions lead to physical dissection of the eyes.

At the time when the early texts of *The Inner Canon of the Yellow Thearch* were being compiled, the first individual descriptions of pharmaceutical drugs were developing into an independent *Běncǎo* (本草) literature. The oldest of these works, the "Shén Nóng's Canon on Materia Medica" (神农本草经 *Shén nóng běn cǎo jīng*) from about the 1st century A.D., enumerates at least seven substances with ophthalmological effects. Most of these drugs were said to brighten "dulled eyes," while others were recommended for "green blindness," "red painful eyes," "tearing," "red-white membrane in the eye," and other complaints.

References to surgical operations on the eye are found not in the earliest medical writings, but in the general historical literature of the first half of the 1st millennium A.D. Such operations may have been the result of Indian influence, and were performed occasionally, but were never developed as part of regular Chinese medicine. This applies in particular to the Indian method of excising cataracts.

Cataract operations in China can be traced back to the Táng. Astonishingly, the Indian and Buddhist context of these therapeutic procedures was never lost over the following centuries. Ophthalmological literature discussed technical variants of and the instruments used in the cataract excisions, but did not become clearer and better informed over the centuries. Quite the reverse, the most accurate descriptions of the procedures are those of the Táng. In later centuries, written instructions suggest that authors were describing a technique they were personally unfamiliar with. Since cataract excisions in China have been practiced in the traditional way down to the present, the deficient knowledge of the texts may indicate that practitioners of folk medicine mastered the technique and handed it down from generation to generation, while learned medicine distanced itself from such techniques much as it did in Europe, where well into the 19th century the removal of cataracts was an operation one could expect to see being performed at annual fairs, not one performed by university-educated physicians.

3. The eye as an indicator of an internal state

Learned medicine of the Chinese upper classes directed its attention almost exclusively to an internal interpretation of ophthalmological problems. When in the year A.D. 610, the first specialist work on etiology appeared, it became clear what knowledge had developed in the meantime. The eyes were first and foremost considered to be an "indication" (候 *hòu*) of internal states. A total of 51 different eye ailments were traced to a wide variety of different underlying pathologies, as the following example shows.

> When [the light of the] eyes grows dark (目黑 *mù hēi*), then the cause lies in a lack [of qì] in the liver. The eyes are where the essence of the organs manifests, and are the external indicator of [the state of] the liver. The liver stores blood. When the organs are affected by a depletion harm (虛損 *xū sǔn*), blood and qì are insufficient. Consequently, the liver suffers from depletion and cannot nourish the eyes. Hence, [the eyes] cannot distinguish light and darkness. Hence, [the light of] the eyes is darkened.
>
> *Zhū Bìng Yuán Hòu Lùn*, ch. 28, 10

The same text also refers to the possibility of eye diseases of congenital origin and attributable to direct action of exogenous influences. It provided the first detailed description of the etiology of the cataracts.

In the following centuries, ophthalmology continued to develop. The doctrine of systematic correspondences was always the basis of internal interpretations of an increasing number of nosologies. Ailments of the eye which were not interpreted in this way, remained without any theoretical adornment. Sūn Sīmiǎo (孙思邈, 581–682?) wrote, for example, that reading in the moonlight, copying books for many years, and frequent looking into the sun could cause eye troubles. Neither he nor any other writer in the following centuries offered any opinion as to what pathological mechanism could explain these observations.

With the separate development of empirical knowledge and theoretical foundations, the pharmaceutical treatment of eye diseases grew increasingly complex. On the one hand, prescription works recommended formulas which, obviously following theoretical considerations, addressed specific eye problems by treating one or more internal organs. On the other hand, there was a broad spectrum of what may have been empirically substantiated methods of treating the eye directly, including eye drops, lotions for washing the eyes, medicinal washes and steam baths, as well as hot and cold poultices. For a highly educated man like Sūn Sīmiǎo, it was out of the question to recommend curses, say, for night blindness.

The prescription works of Sūn Sīmiǎo are the first texts containing the names of individual points on the skin, where needling was presumed effective for ophthalmological indications such as pain and itching in the pupil, nearsightedness, and night blindness. Interestingly, the mentioning of these standard points hints at the prevalence of so-called prescription acupuncture, which is rated poorly in Western acupuncture literature. In contrast to "true acupuncture," which thinks out a needling strategy on the basis of functional relationships and the conduit system within the body in order to treat an individual problem, prescription acupuncture uses the same points for the same condition, without concern for the condition of the individual patient.

Chinese ophthalmology received new etiological stimuli for its development when at the beginning of the 12th century different schools of thought postulated different ideas about basic etiological factors. Liú Wánsù (刘完素, 1110–1200), for example, had arrived at the conviction that all diseases were the result of excessive heat in the body, so that all therapeutic interventions should be geared to cooling. Consequently, he wrote a text whose agenda the title made explicit, that "all unclear vision, reddening and swellings, and membranes affecting the eyes are due to heat."

Lǐ Gǎo (李杲, 1180–1251) attributed the overwhelming majority of diseases including eye troubles to disturbance of stomach function. He was therefore the first author not to mention the previously exalted significance of the liver in the etiology of eye diseases.

Neither of these two, nor other conceptions could achieve general acceptance; the heterogeneous theoretical background characteristic of Chinese medicine is also seen in ophthalmology. No authority prescribed for later clinicians or writers which direction future developments should take. Each person was—and is—free to scoop from the rich fund of historical opinion whatever suited his personal conviction, and thereby claim legitimacy for his work.

4. The *Yín Hǎi Jīng Wēi*

The heights that the development of Chinese ophthalmology reached can be seen in a work such as the *Yín Hǎi Jīng Wēi* (银海精微, "Essential Subtleties on the Silver Sea"). This work, probably from the 15th century, now available in English translation for readers without knowledge of the Chinese language, contains the full spectrum of theoretical and practical knowledge of traditional Chinese ophthalmology.

No small part of the 81 nosographies of the *Yín Hǎi Jīng Wēi* can be interpreted from the point of view of modern ophthalmology; many descriptions of eye problems by the Chinese authors are so detailed that correspondences to quite specific modern diagnostic categories can be posited or suggested.

The following text under the heading of "epidemic red eye," for example, can barely be interpreted as referring to anything but epidemic keratoconjunctivitis:

> [The term] 'epidemic red eye' refers to the ability of poisonous qì flowing between heaven and earth to spread among the people. If one person's eyes

> are affected, that person will spread it to the entire family; all, regardless of whether they are adults or children, will be affected once. [...] [Its symptoms of] swelling, pain, sandy roughness, and difficulty opening [the eyes] will be cured after about five days. [...] Hence, the illness comes to rest [after this period]. [...] Even though the swellings and pain may be severe, the black part of the eye and pupil will not be harmed in the end.

The epidemic nature of the disease, its degree of infectiousness, the fact that any person is only "affected once," thereby gaining lifelong immunity, and finally the local symptoms are described in a language that makes them easily understandable to clinicians of contemporary biomedicine.

The overwhelming majority of therapies of the *Yīn Hǎi Jīng Wēi* are based on internal and topical application of pharmaceutical prescriptions. In many cases, the nature of the disease also called for petty-surgical interventions, mostly with the aim of opening blood vessels or excising excrescences. The excision of cataracts was prescribed together with Buddhist prayers, but for reasons previously mentioned, there is considerable room for doubt about the competence of the author.

Subsequent to the publication of the *Yīn Hǎi Jīng Wēi*, traditional Chinese ophthalmology received no fundamental impetus for further development. Individual authors expressed their views on one minor problem or another, yet the theoretical framework and the spectrum of therapeutic interventions underwent no further change. In recent times (the 1990's), texts have appeared in the People's Republic of China that integrate the historical development of Chinese ophthalmology with the official modern interpretation of Chinese medicine; insofar as traditional notions are not religiously founded, do not appear absurd from the modern point of view, and are free of health-damaging clinical consequences, they are preserved and brought as far as possible into harmony with modern medical knowledge.

CHAPTER FIVE
USE OF DRUGS AND PHARMACOLOGY

1. The validity of systematic correspondence

Historical consideration of traditional Chinese ophthalmology directs attention to one important, if not central, question in the evaluation of Chinese medicine, namely the relationship between theory and practice. This question touches on the comprehensive validity of the doctrines of yīn and yáng and the five phases.

Ancient Chinese physicians distinguished between eye diseases that arose from external causes or hazardous use of the eyes, such as reading without sufficient illumination, and others attributed to the consequences of internal disturbances. The theoretical foundations of traditional Chinese medicine, as we have already stated, were only applied in the latter category of diseases.

The doctrines of systematic correspondence were not adduced to clarify why reading without sufficient light damages the eyesight; nor were they adduced to explain the infectiousness of a particular ailment, or how in certain cases a patient once affected could gain life immunity. In the wealth of medical theory literature that accumulated over the imperial age, we know of no texts whose authors reflected on the selective theoretical elucidation of problems of this sort. We can therefore offer no statement as to whether the doctrines of yīn and yáng and the five phases were unsuited to incorporating such problems, or whether such problems were quite simply not considered by the writers in question to be worthy of theoretical substantiation.

Indications as to the validity of traditional theories are found only by considering numerous facets of Chinese medicine. The history of leprosy in China, for instance, suggests that systematic correspondence may have been hard pressed to explain real pathological processes. For over a thousand years, the description of afflictions that closely fit the modern definition of leprosy were left unexplained by yīn-yáng and five-phase theories. In the 14th century, finally, two authors in quick succession attempted to incorporate all the possible manifestations of this disease that had been observed over the centuries into a framework of systematic correspondence. Their promptings were not taken up by subsequent writers, and leprosy—or those afflictions that either actually constitute leprosy or that take a similar course—was left, after a short interlude of theorization, to a purely pragmatic approach and treated with pharmaceutical procedures, without apparent need of theoretical underpinning.

Given the dominance of the doctrines of theoretical correspondence since Chinese antiquity in explaining the physiological and pathological processes in the healthy and afflicted organism, the comparison with leprosy suggests that yīn-yáng and five-phase theories preserved their validity over two millennia essentially in areas that lay beyond empirical scrutiny and that, unlike leprosy or blindness, cannot be regarded as transculturally valid realities.

Such transculturally valid realities can be seen in certain functions of drugs, that is, in all pharmacological effects that bring about tangible or visible changes in physical states. Whether a substance reduces a fever, produces diarrhea, or relieves a headache can be empirically demonstrated and—unlike "kidney yáng weakness"—is not a cultural construct. The cultural explanation of the effects of drugs are, therefore, a further test case for the validity of traditional Chinese doctrines.

2. The theoretical substantiation of drug effects

Surprisingly, historical analysis shows that in China two medical traditions were practiced without any mutual contact (with the exception of one author in the 3rd century A.D.) for an almost unimaginably long period of 1,500 years. On the one hand, there was the medicine of systematic correspondences using needle therapy and dietetics fed on the yīn-yáng and five-phase theories, and on the other, the pharmaceutical healing tradition, which attempted to harness the effects of drugs to relieve innumerable manifestations of disease without recourse to the laws of systematic correspondence.

The medicine of systematic correspondence defines internal afflictions in terms of yīn-yáng and five-phase doctrines as "kidney yáng weakness," to take up once more an example already mentioned, and makes it a central concern that each patient should be seen as an individual problem. In contrast, the pharmaceutical prescription literature of China applied, in almost the same way as modern Western medicine, label-like disease concepts such as "fever" or *nüè* (malaria), which were imposed on patients without consideration of their age, constitution, or sex and which required treatment largely independent of their individual conditions.

It was only beginning with the 12th century A.D. that the situation in the general history of ideas led to an approximation of the two lines of tradition. A thousand years earlier, in European antiquity, Galen had linked the empirically highly developed medicine of the eastern Mediterranean with theories that had previously been limited to interpreting etiological, physiological, and pathological processes in the body, thereby creating the first European pharmacology in the sense of a stringent theory explaining the way drugs affect the body. With very similar goals, Chinese medical scholars from the end of the Sòng attempted to create a pharmacology based on systematic correspondence.

The problem facing the Chinese writers was largely identical with Galen's. On the one hand, there was a refined theory available, and on the other, a rich body of pharmaceutical knowledge. In China, the theory to which drugs were to be linked was obviously that of the doctrines of systematic correspondence.

Since antiquity, the qualities of edible substances had been determined by their flavor and temperature. In theoretical literature, these qualities had been discussed as abstractions and in their their significance for dietetics. *The Inner Canon of the Yellow Thearch* states, "In the case of a heat disease, cooling (清 *qīng*) is used; in a cold disease, heat is used." In contrast, the materia medica literature referred to the flavor and temperature of drugs only to identify them.

In the late Sòng, authors forged a bridge between the flavor and temperature qualities of particular drugs on the one hand and the effects of these qualities in the organism on the other.

Flavor was defined as a yīn quality and temperature a yáng quality. Warm, hot, and balanced temperatures of a drug were considered strong qualities and hence as yáng in yáng; cold and cool temperatures were considered weak qualities, and hence yīn in yáng. Sour, bitter, and salty were considered to be strong flavor qualities and rated as yīn in yīn; acrid, sweet, and neutral were interpreted as weak flavor qualities, and therefore characterized as yáng in yīn.

In this way, scholars postulated for the first time that particular drugs and drug effects empirically defined in terms of yīn and yáng, i.e., heating (a yáng-in-yáng effect), dispersion (a yīn-in-yáng effect), draining (a yīn-in-yīn effect), and penetration (a yáng-in-yīn effect), had certain affinities with yīn or yáng categorizations of the organs, particular diseases, or the time (day or night) when drugs were effective.

Flavor and temperature qualities of drugs were of course also categorized according to the five phases. Salty taste and warm temperature were seen as qualities of wood, sour taste and hot temperature as qualities of fire, sweet taste and balanced temperature as qualities of earth, bitter taste and cool temperature as qualities of metal, and acrid taste and cold temperature as qualities of water. In this way, certain affinities were established, in particular for the functional spheres categorized according to the five phases, i.e., liver and gallbladder (wood), heart and small

intestine (fire), spleen and stomach (earth), lung and large intestine (metal), and the kidney and bladder (water).

Many authors derived the effects of a drug directly from
its flavor quality without recourse to the yīn-yáng categories.
They were convinced that acrid substances dissipate and promote movement, that bitter substances drain and dry, and sweet
substances supplement and moisten, that sour substances as-
tringe and prevent or halt the flow of fluids, that salty substances clean and soften, and that substances of neutral flavor
drain dampness and disinhibit urination.

Agreement between all writers on the evaluation of drug qualities was never achieved, and possibly never even sought. *The
Inner Canon of the Yellow Thearch*, for example, identified acrid
and sweet as yáng and therefore as dissipating, sour and bitter as
yīn and therefore draining, and neutral flavor also draining but
as yáng. Similarly in partial contrast to later categorizations,
The Inner Canon of the Yellow Thearch established: "Sour flavor enters the liver. Acrid flavor enters the lung. Bitter flavor
enters the heart. Salty flavor enters the kidney. Sweet flavor
enters the spleen."

Such differences were never settled. The fact that some writers of the Sòng-Jīn-Yuán period described categorizations other
than those of *The Inner Canon of the Yellow Thearch* did not
affect the authority of this classic. From a Western perspective,
this might seem surprising since the consequences of such contradictions were considerable if the various categorizations had
any effect on the clinical application of drugs. In fact, it is of
course not known whether practitioners actually applied theory
in practice, or whether these categorizations were merely intellectual mind games based on fashionable tendencies of the time.
Probably, the whole theoretical framework that was extended,
mainly by Sòng-Jīn-Yuán scholars, to the use of drugs on the
basis of systematic correspondences was irrelevant since the systematic categorization of organ functions and functional spheres
only rested on ancient speculation.

Possibly because of the differences of opinion between individual authors over the flavor and temperature qualities of individual drugs and hence over the definition of yīn-yáng and five-phase categorizations of individual substances and their effects, Zhāng Yuánsù (张元素, 12th century) completely evaded the problem and attributed functions not to qualities, but directly to particular drugs. He emphasized that the effect of a substance depended on which conduit it entered. This conduit approach gave rise to the notion that particular drugs are capable of leading other substances to specific places in the body and hence of enabling them to produce their effect there. Zhāng Yuánsù also emphasized the effect of drugs on particular organs, stating for example, that *huáng lián* (Rhizoma Coptidis) drained heart fire and that *chuān xiōng* (Radix Ligustici Wallichii) dissipated liver qì.

The association between drugs and organs or particular functions has since become the most important classification of drug action. Liú Wánsù (刘完素, 1110–1200), for example, through the five-phase association that he ascribed to each substance, saw direct relationships between these substances and the possible climatic influences, which penetrate the body from outside and cause damage there. Accordingly, a drug classed as wood is best suited to expelling wind, the evil associated with wood, from the body. No explanation is given anywhere in the literature as to how a principle of "like repels like" comes into play, i.e., why a drug associated with the wood phase should act against wood, rather than having a wood-strengthening effect in the way that heat drugs do not eliminate heat but increase it.

In the 14th and 15th centuries, with the end of historical trends that had favored an approximation between Confucianism and Daoism as much as the approximation between the medicine of systematic correspondence and pharmacy, the search for theoretical understanding of drug effects on the basis of systematic correspondence came to a standstill. No further impetus in this direction followed. Authors and users of the following centuries were free to choose from the various approaches that the Sòng-Jīn-Yuán left for posterity the one that suited them best.

Later developments in the classification of drugs were innovative to a varying degree and centered mostly around empirical effects. In the 18th century, several authors stressed the eight patterns (八法 bā fǎ): sweating (汗 hàn), vomiting (吐 tù), purgation (下 xià), harmonization (和 hé), warming (温 wēn), cooling (清 qīng), and dispersion (消 xiāo).

Characteristic of the poor ability of the premises of systematic correspondence to gain long-term acceptance, and, hence, indicative for an evaluation of the corresponding theories is the enumeration of indications attributed to individual drugs from the dissolution of Sòng-Jīn-Yuán trends to the present. The primary indications of drugs were conditions such as insomnia, poor appetite, uterine bleeding, urine retention, irritability, water accumulations, fatigue, diarrhea, vomiting, and many others. Statements such as "fortifies the spleen," "supplements the middle burner," "warms the kidneys and invigorates yáng," had a rather rhetorical character, unless, as in the case of kidney yáng depletion, for example, they were to be equated with indications. Kidney yáng depletion, for example, is a fixed formula for a syndrome including impotence, spermatorrhea, cold and weak legs, as well as lumbar pain.

3. Pharmaceutical processing of crude drugs

Over the whole of its history, Chinese pharmacy has used both individual drugs for particular afflictions and prescriptions composed of several substances. The arsenal of drugs, which over the last two millennia has continually been developed and has been published in a variety of monographs and prescription literature, is very impressive. In terms of the variety of content and the scope of the text, the *Běn Cǎo Gāng Mù* (本草纲目) ("Materia Medica Arranged According to Drug Descriptions and Technical Aspects") represents the acme of materia medica literature. This work, compiled by Lǐ Shízhēn (李时珍, 1518–1593)

and published posthumously in the year 1596, contains detailed descriptions of over 1,800 different drugs.

The oldest extant prescription text, the *Wŭ Shí Èr Bìng Fāng* (五十二病方), "Prescriptions for 52 Diseases," unearthed from the Măwángduī tomb, which was sealed in 167 B.C., indicates that a refined pharmaceutical technology had already developed by this time. The methods for the collection and processing of crude substances from plants, animals, and minerals, and their preparation into a variety of drug forms, that by the time of the Măwángduī text had already reached a high level, were continuously further developed over the centuries, as testified by not only special technical literature, but also general materia medica and prescription texts.

From antiquity, Chinese pharmacy held the notion, which is intelligible from a modern viewpoint, that drugs from particular geographical regions showed better effects than the same drugs from other regions. The development of a drug's effects was seen in conjunction with general processes of maturation in the course of a year. Literature instructed pharmacists that the subterranean medicinal parts of plants should be harvested before they reached full maturity and their strength moved to the upper areas of the plant. Flowers were to be harvested before they opened, the whole plant in later summer or autumn.

Apart from the mechanical methods such as grating, pulverizing, and cutting, drug-processing methods largely made use of water and heating to enhance or modify the known pharmaceutical effects. The most commonly used processes used today are as follows:

1. *zhēng* 蒸, steaming, followed by sun-drying.

2. *zhŭ* 煮, boiling in clear water, rice water, liquor, vinegar, boy's urine, or other liquids.

3. *áo* 熬, reducing a decoction to a syrup.

4. *zhì* 炙, roasting with fluids. Roasting with wine increases the ability of a substance to open blocks in the conduits, relieve pain, and dispel wind. Roasting with ginger juice decreases the tendency of certain cold bitter drugs to irritate the stomach. Roasting with vinegar enhances the astringent and pain-relieving abilities of certain substances.

5. *pào* 炮, brief heating to a high temperature until brown. This method reduces poisonous constituents.

6. *chǎo* 炒, stir-frying. With salt, it directs the effect of the drug to the kidney.

7. *hōng* 烘, slow drying of flowers and insects.

4. The preparation of drug forms

Drugs processed in any of the various ways usually have to be transformed into drug forms in a further stage before they can be taken. The most common form is decoction in water, and less often in other fluids. Different instructions are given in the literature as to the duration of decoction and size of flame; there are numerous possibilities of varying the decoction process for different drugs.

Powders, pills, and pastes of Chinese pharmacy are similar in their preparation and their purposes to corresponding drug forms in traditional European pharmacy. In their applications, however, there are some significant differences. For example, "point ointments" are unknown in European pharmacy. These are pharmaceutical preparations in ointment or paste form, which are supposed to be able to produce very different effects on the body depending on which acupuncture points they are applied to.

5. The synergism and hierarchy of drugs in prescriptions

The earliest pharmaceutical literature from the first centuries A.D. captures the experience of doctors in the simultaneous administration of different substances. Seven social metaphors serve the description of the seven possible interactions between substances within one formula:

1. *xiāng xū* 相须, "one helps the other," means the mutual enhancement of similar effects of different drugs when administered together.

2. *xiāng shǐ* 相使, "one endows the other," means the mutual enhancement of different actions of different drugs when administered together.

3. *xiāng wèi* 相畏, "one fears the other," the reduction of undesired effects of a drug by another drug with which it is administered.

4. *xiāng shā* 相杀, "one kills the other," the elimination of undesired effects of a drug through another drug with which it is administered.

5. *xiāng wù* 相恶, "one hates the other," means the mutual reduction of desired effects of different drugs when administered together.

6. *xiāng fǎn* 相反, "one clashes with the other," means producing undesired new effects through simultaneous administration of different drugs that are not produced when the drugs are administered individually.

7. *dān xíng* 单行, "one goes alone," means administering a single drug without being influenced by other drugs administered simultaneously.

Metaphorical names are also given to hierarchies of substances within a prescription. The main constituent of a prescription, from antiquity to the early years of communist China, was called the "ruler" (君 jūn). In the cultural revolution, writers substituted the word zhǔ 主 from zhǔ xí 主席, "chairman." The "sovereign," or "chairman," is responsible for the therapeutic aim of the formula. He is flanked by several "ministers" (臣 chén), or, since the cultural revolution, "assistants" (辅 fǔ), which support the effects of the ruler. Furthermore, a balanced formula has a number of "helpers" (佐 zuǒ), who provide various services: they may serve to soften the strength of the main drug, or help the sovereign/chairman and ministers/assistants by, for example, supporting the cooling main drug of a prescription with a warming action. Finally, there are the "messengers," who either have a calming, harmonizing effect, or serve as conductor drugs ensuring that the expected effect of the other substances reaches the desired place.

6. Proprietary drugs and individual preparation

Like their European counterparts, Chinese physicians in antiquity recognized that certain substances or combinations of substances always have the same effect on different patients with the same affliction. At least since the 13th century, China has had a broad network for the manufacture and marketing of ready-to-use drugs. In Europe, the same development took place in the 19th century with the rise of the pharmaceutical industry, which is now a major component of the health-care system. Not least, marketing strategies with the aim of customer retention, product loyalty, and corporate identity point to clear parallels between the procedures of Chinese producers of traditional proprietary drugs over the last centuries and the advertising methods of the modern pharmaceutical industry.

Alongside proprietary medicines, there has, since the Sòng-Jīn-Yuán period, existed the desideratum derived from the doctrines of systematic correspondence to examine the personal condition of each patient and design a prescription accordingly. This approach was restricted socially to the level of educated physicians who applied the theoretical premises of systematic correspondence consistently in drug therapy. Their intentions were served best by decoctions. The need posed by the theories to reevaluate the condition of the patient as far as possible every day and the individual consideration of different patients even when presenting similar disease conditions call for frequent adjustment of the constituents of a prescription to address depletion or repletion, blockages or excessive flows. The dose of a decoction is always that required for one day; the composition of the prescription can be altered the following day.

7. Modern research

Drug therapy has been the focus of Chinese medicine for over two thousand years, especially in the treatment of acute conditions. Countless substances have been tried over the centuries, and, for reasons seldom clear today, adopted into the arsenal of drugs. The encounter with Western science in the 20th century has led to a scientific investigation of drug effects.

Many drugs have been found to contain pharmacologically active agents. The question as to whether the effects that can be demonstrated today are the same as those postulated in the past has only rarely received a satisfactory answer. Particularly problematic and largely unresolved is the question as to how to evaluate traditional prescriptions. Modern pharmacology possesses all the possibilities to investigate the constituents of individual substances and the mechanisms of their effects, but the synergistic effects of combinations of several substances create difficulties.

For decades Western drug companies have conducted large-scale screening programs to investigate China's arsenal of materia medica in search of new drugs for Western medicine. However, barely a handful of Chinese drugs have found their way into modern medicine, the most important of these being *má huáng*, *Ephedra sinica* Staph., from which ephedrine is extracted.

Also for decades, countless Chinese and Japanese investigations have been made to determine the effect of traditional formulas. The methods used in these studies are rarely in keeping with the strict requirements of modern pharmacological research. As a result, reports regularly appearing in the Chinese press of drugs being "over 90% effective" defy unequivocal interpretation, and so far have not led to any enrichment of the international pharmacopoeia to speak of. Despite this, a large number of traditional drug producers in China manufacture proprietary brands for sale at home and worldwide to a receptive clientèle of largely Asiatic origin.

Chapter Six
Chinese Medicine in China in the Modern Era and Present

1. The political context

Traditional Chinese medicine in China exists no longer as an independent healing system with its own ideas and practices. The loss of the not only conceptual but also diagnostic and therapeutic independence is the result of a policy of the People's Republic of China geared to this end. It is also, however, the result of a long historical process, whose causes were present long before encounters with the West.

Just as the traditional political world view lost its unity from the 17th century and crumbled into numerous individual views that the various schools of thought recommended to solve the many political problems of the Chinese empire, so Chinese medicine after the end of the age of Sòng neo-Confucianism never again recovered any kind of unity. The splintering into various etiological and therapeutic principles that had begun in the 12th century continued in the Míng and Qīng.

When Western medicine was systematically and extensively introduced into China by Protestant missionaries at the beginning of the 19th century, it did not encounter a homogenous system, but a disparate conglomerate of very different ideas and practices characterized in part by systematic correspondence, in part by speculation and superstition, in part by religious doctrines, and in part by the experience and economic interests of wandering healers.

Western medicine was immediately convincing at least to Chinese doctors who were willing to learn. Quite a number of representatives of traditional medicine who were denied access to

Western medicine expressed themselves defensively for obvious reasons. For Chinese doctors and students who had the possibility to get to grips with the theory of Western medicine from the end of the 19th century, there opened a world that was both familiar and new.

What seemed familiar to the Chinese was the new bacteriological view that had recently swiftly risen to dominance. The demonological healing of China with its notions of evil powers, which, taking no account of the moral condition of their victims, penetrated the body to cause damage there, could easily be likened to the modern Western notions of pathogenic agents, as could the naturalistic medicine of China, which was based on the notion of "evils," which in various forms "occupy" the body, move within it, and settle at a particular spot where they then give rise to disease and which have either to be killed or driven out if the patient is to be cured. Chinese pharmacy had overcome the short theorising interlude of the Sòng-Jīn-Yuán period and had returned to an empiricism that was hardly any different from the direct symptom-medicament relationship of European medicine.

The only thing that was new for Chinese men of medicine was Western medicine's belief in progress. Science seeks fulfillment in a future golden age; traditional medicine, including traditional Chinese medicine, always proceeds from the assumption that the golden age of medicine lies in the past. The basic cultural challenge in China's encounter was that of exchanging the authority of antiquity for faith in an as-yet-unwritten future. The fact that this challenge presented no insuperable obstacles is shown by the first decades of the encounter, when all social forces committed to China's renewal considered Western science and technology alone to offer a way forward, and were prepared to make room for traditional Chinese medicine only in memory of the "bankrupt feudal age" of the empire.

Nobody in the West wishing to assess traditional Chinese medicine as inadequate could find such hostile and hurtful words for this form of medicine as came from the full spectrum of political decision-makers and reformist or even revolutionary intellectuals of the first two or three decades of the 20th century in China. The nationalist forces united in the Guómíngdǎng (Kuomintang, KMT) as well as the communists since that time were acting in accordance with political, economic, and social pressures when they appeared to give up their reservations about Chinese medicine. In actual fact, neither of these two forces, one of which rules only in Taiwan and the other holding political responsibility for the mainland, has ever accorded traditional Chinese medicine a future as an equal alternative to modern Western medicine, even if the rhetoric on the mainland might at first sight suggest the opposite.

The general neglect of traditional Chinese medicine in Taiwan over the last decades corresponds in mainland China to the gradual and inescapable infiltration of the old corpus of ideas with those of modern science. Just as the PRC government is effecting the transition from the socialist planned economy to the capitalist market economy not abruptly, but with skillful long-term planning, it has chosen to deal with the question of traditional medicine not by confrontation, but by modest change.

2. Phases of change

Traditional Chinese medicine is comparable with a tree that has lost its roots. The wood is still available and can be put to many meaningful uses, yet nourishment and further development no longer spring from its own forces. Chinese medicine has been in this situation since it lost the philosophical and political environment that had once given it plausibility and acceptance and allowed it to survive for two thousand years.

It was not clinical validity that gave the conceptual construct of Chinese medicine its longevity, but its abiding plausibility. In Europe, the frequent changes in medical systems from the beginnings of medicine in Greek antiquity were the result of frequent fundamental changes and shifts in sociopolitical and philosophical conditions. Greek city states, Hellenism, the Roman empire, late antiquity and early middle ages, high middle ages, Renaissance, the pre-modern, and modern age replaced each other every three to four hundred years. They created diachronic and synchronic upheavals in existential conditions, which deeply influenced the view of the body and sickness.

In China, by constrast, the basic framework remained largely the same over the whole of the imperial age, irrespective of any internal dynamics. The changes within this basic framework, as seen in the era of Sòng neo-Confucianism, left their marks on Chinese medicine, but were incapable of changing its fundamental features.

It was the encounter with the West that prompted the first basic questioning. In the beginning, a small number of medical reformers who were defenders of Chinese culture deluded themselves in the belief that the adoption of Western techniques and drugs would suffice to give Chinese medicine new strength. Táng Zōnghǎi (唐宗海, 1862–1918), Máo Jǐngyì (毛景义, fl. end of Qīng) and others made comparisons between Chinese and Western medicine, and pointed the way into the future with symbioses of various kinds. The aim of their plans was to ensure the enduring dominance of Chinese medicine. A product of this era was the catch-phrase "Chinese medicine treats the root; Western medicine treats the symptom," which is still occasionally to be heard to this day.

From the 1930's on, the direction changed. The few writers who thought about how Chinese medicine could be saved began to see thorough-going scientific research as the only possibility of wresting meaningful and still usable elements from what was evidently a medley of viable and outmoded ideas and practices. This approach is the program that has been followed by the Chinese communists, with a short interruption during the Cultural Revolution. It sees on the horizon a scientifically founded medicine in which as many elements of traditional Chinese medicine as possible are to be included.

Development in this direction requires no force; it comes of its own accord. Each new generation in China finds the ancient philosophies increasingly alien. The doctrines of yīn and yáng and the five phases have lost their rank as the obvious way of understanding reality; they are no longer part of school or family education, and have to be painstakingly learned. The medicine these doctrines serve is today cognitively isolated. In contrast, the modern sciences and technology, physics, and mathematics are part of the education of every Chinese child. They have made their imprint over the whole of private and professional life, making modern medicine automatically, as it were, appear to be true.

3. Administrative measures

Quite a few countries of the third world have attempted to enter the modern world by prohibiting traditional healing practices. The government of the People's Republic of China has taken a different path. It has instituted a series of measures that have supported the inevitable dominance of Western medicine. It has taken the wind out of the traditionalists' sails by giving them far-reaching equal rights in the command of diagnostic and therapeutic techniques and drugs. It propagates the existence of the three paths, that is, allowing modern medicine to develop according to its own laws, allowing traditional Chinese medicine to seek its own development, and where meaningful and possible, allowing the two systems to be combined.

Chinese medicine is allowed to seek its "own development," but not without guidance. An unending succession of regulations has meant that the term "Chinese medicine" refers no longer to the tradition in its former entirety, but to a small fragment of it that from the modern viewpoint clashes neither with scientific knowledge nor with Marxism's rejection of any remaining elements of feudalism and metaphysics.

Volker Scheid, an ethnologist who is intimately acquainted with the practice of Chinese medicine, has shown, through the example of changes in the treatment of stroke, the subtle way in which Western concepts have influenced Chinese medicine, possibly even before the 20th century. As the name *zhòng fēng* (中风), "struck by wind," which is still used to this day, suggests, stroke was interpreted in Chinese antiquity as being caused by wind. With the propagation of various etiological principles through diverging schools since the late Sòng, attention shifted to what is called "internal wind," which, however it arose, was to be eliminated from the body. Perhaps as a result of the Western association between stroke and blood circulation, Chinese writers at the end of the Qīng Dynasty were explaining stroke in terms of the traditional concepts of "blood stasis" and were recommending substances from Chinese pharmacy which since time immemorial had been accorded "blood-quickening" or "stasis-dispelling" effects.

While quite a few Western adherents of traditional Chinese medicine in Europe and the USA reject any relationship between the Chinese concept of *xuè* (血) and the notion of blood in Western medicine, and either refuse to translate *xuè* as blood or, at least in English, write it with a capital letter to highlight the fact the Chinese understand something entirely different by blood than Westerners do, such scruples are unknown in China. Although the Chinese are well aware that antiquity assigned the blood other properties and functions than the modern age does, this does not prevent ancient statements about the blood from being interpreted in a new way, and the whole gamut of hematological diagnosis and therapy of modern medicine from being carried over to Chinese medicine and vice-versa.

Every textbook published in China on Chinese medicine contains an introduction to the doctrines of systematic correspondence, yet the research on Chinese medicine that has been demanded by the government is based only on modern scientific methodology.

In 1995, the Gānsù Province Science and Technology Press published *A Practical Manual of Combined Chinese and Western Medicine.* The editor responsible for the book, the vice-director of the Medical Academy of Gānsù, and a nationally recognized authority on the integration of Chinese and Western medicine, presented in the book the findings of studies conducted over a period of thirty years. A key point in his recommendations is that a condition should be diagnosed on the basis of Western procedures, and if necessary treated using traditional Chinese medical methods and drugs. The book contains a long list of internal diseases with Western diagnostic parameters and the correspondences in traditional terminology.

The effect of such advice on actual practice cannot be foreseen. Over the past decades in China, as in other countries where a population enjoys the choice between modern and traditional medicine, a relatively stable pattern of demand by patients has formed. Traditional medical care is sought particularly by patients with chronic diseases that from the Western medical viewpoint are resistant to treatment. The general preference for Western medicine which is today also found in China as in other countries rests on factors of time and economy.

The book published in Gānsù furnishes evidence, however, of how traditional medicine is gradually being encircled by modern science. Therapeutic techniques, above all acupuncture, are being increasingly removed from their traditional background and integrated into modern medicine. In 1982, the Chinese government commissioned the compilation of a catalog of pharmaceutical raw materials in China, which was to contain all substances of animal, vegetable, and mineral origin used as drugs in traditional Chinese medicine. After ten years, the catalogue listed more than 11,000 plants, 1,500 animals, 80 minerals, and a list of some 100,000 applications and prescriptions.

In 1986, the government promulgated a law for the management of traditional Chinese pharmacy, which laid down standards for the identification of Chinese medicinal plants and gave each plant a specific name with a view to solving the problem of different names for the same substances in many parts of the country and that of different substances having the same name.

On January 1, 1995, uniform criteria for diagnosis and efficacy in traditional Chinese medicine were introduced. All institutions of teaching and scientific research are to apply the new standards. Since the name and explanations of traditional concepts were also included in English, this enactment points to a bid by the Chinese authorities to influence the international development of Chinese medicine. The standardized terminology is supposed to facilitate scientific and economic exchange.

Also in 1995, a committee for medical science composed of experts of traditional Chinese medicine and members of the Department of Medical Research of the British Wellcome Institute was formed. The aim of the committee is apparently to promote research between Chinese scientists of traditional Chinese medicine and researchers of the Wellcome Institute in the field of medicine and pharmacology.

One measure after another serves to integrate traditional medicine into modern medicine and to create an unmistakably Chinese variant of modern medicine, which with an extended diagnostic and therapeutic framework, is hoped will be more attractive than "pure" Western medicine and hence marketable worldwide. In 1994, China's exports to Europe and the USA of proprietary drugs of Chinese medicine reached a total value of US $400 million; and as the president of the National Administration of Chinese Medicine stated in 1995, a yearly increase of 5 percent is expected.

4. Prospects

Chinese medicine has lost its original roots and consequently its modern clinical practice has largely forfeited its conceptual independence. That does not of course mean that Chinese medicine as a cultural heritage will disappear in China.

First, the historical knowledge accumulated over the course of the centuries and contained in an extremely varied literature is preserved to the extent that the literature is still available. The number of pre-1911 titles is estimated to be 13,000 to 15,000. Facsimile copies of pre-Republic original texts as well as more or less carefully edited and commented new editions of old texts, which Chinese publishers are putting out in ever larger numbers, provide for the unforeseeable future inexhaustible ground for a whole variety of research.

Second, the PRC government supports efforts to preserve the knowledge of older doctors. In October 1990, the authorities selected 700 young doctors to enter an apprenticeship of several years to 464 renowned veteran specialists of Chinese medicine. In October 1994, a first group of 600 of apprentices finished their course, and it was immediately announced that a further 500 known old Chinese doctors should assist with the training of future generations of practitioners. Although there is no guarantee that the older physicians are willing to fully initiate younger doctors assigned to them by the state in all aspects of their skills, these initiatives at least document the attempt to save what can still be saved.

Present-day practice in China is characterized by great variety, much as it probably was in past centuries. Although the state is at pains to guide development in a particular direction, doctors espouse all manner of interpretations of old and new approaches. To this extent, it is quite justifiable to assert that the tree of Chinese medicine is still alive and will continue to live on. This is only possible because it draws the strength needed for adaptation from another root, i.e., from a new system of thought.

Chapter Seven
The Long March West

In the historic change in Chinese politics in 1976, relations between China and the West began anew and swiftly increased in intensity. This gave Westerners interested in Chinese medicine previously almost unimaginable opportunities to see Chinese medicine in practice in China itself. Countless laypeople, healers, and physicians have taken advantage of the new situation to gain knowledge and practical skills in China and apply them to patients in their homeland on their return. In the meanwhile, national societies and private training centers have sprung up in all Western countries to meet the requirements of the increasing professionalization of these groups.

At the same time, Western interest in acupuncture and traditional drug therapy has stimulated efforts in China itself to sell Chinese medicine to Europe and the USA. Chinese practitioners with very different qualifications practice in all Western countries, making incomes that with their abilities they could never make in China itself. Manufacturers of traditional pharmaceutical products in China and Japan are developing strategies to market their products on the international markets, and the Chinese authorities are contributing by steering the reception of acupuncture in the West along lines that suit their interests.

With all these developments, it is easy to forget that the attention Western physicians are now paying Chinese medicine is merely another high point in an interaction between the two bodies of medicine that has been going on for a long time.

At least since the time William of Rubruk described his *Journey to the Land of the Mongols* between 1253 and 1255, news of China's own medicine reached Europe again and again. Marco Polo (1254–1324) reported on the "famous natural doctors who knew all the secrets of nature." Details about the nature of Far Eastern medicine however, were first provided by Europeans who spent longer periods in China, Japan, and Indonesia, and for various different reasons fastened their attention on healing, thereby gaining the opportunity to acquire a broader knowledge.

1. Portuguese Jesuits

Since the beginning of the 16th century, Jesuit missionaries from Portugal were trying to establish a foothold in East Asia. The Chinese authorities showed no interest in such contacts and turned the foreigners away; some neighboring countries, though, were more open, at least in the beginning. In 1549, the Jesuits were given permission to set up missions in Japan. The combination of missionary and medical activity proved especially helpful in convincing Japanese natives of the sense and value of the Christian doctrine. Consequently, Portuguese doctors practiced together with converted Japanese doctors in hospitals and leper colonies. Thus they inevitably had a chance to acquaint themselves with the Japanese variant of Chinese medicine.

For this reason, it is not surprising that the earliest reports about acupuncture and moxibustion from East Asia reached Europe in a letter from a Portuguese priest to an abbot in Coimbra: "In general, the Japanese are very healthy because of the climate, which is very temperate and healthy, because they eat little and because they do not drink clear water (fresh, unboiled water), the cause of so many diseases. When they fall ill, it is their custom in all diseases to stick silver needles into the abdomen, arms, and back, etc. At the same time they use fire buttons made of herbs."

What are here described as "fire buttons" are clearly the small balls of mugwort floss that the Japanese burnt on many spots of the body surface, much to the astonishment of European eyewitnesses. In a *Vocabulario da Lingoa de Iapam* ("Vocabulary of the Language of Japan"), published by the Jesuit college in Nagasaki in 1603, the herbal preparation used in this kind of cauterization was first given the name *mogusa*; in the year 1679, a book entitled *Het Podagra* on the subject of gout by the minister Hermann Buschof (died 1674) introduced the term "moxa," which is still commonly used today, for the cones of mugwort used in moxibustion. During a long stay in Batavia (now Djakarta), Buschof, having experienced the healing effects of moxa, that is moxibustion, on his own condition of gout, learned the technique and used it in the treatment of other patients.

The dictionaries compiled by the Portuguese Jesuits in Japan also provide a useful index of early knowledge about acupuncture. The Japanese-Latin Lexicon of 1595 included eight entries on acupuncture and moxibustion; the *Vocabulario* of 1603 includes 50 terms for various needles made of different metals and various techniques by which needles were inserted by turning or tapping.

The missionaries did not only learn about the practical aspects of Sino-Japanese medicine; the dictionaries show that they also strove to penetrate the philosophical foundations of this medicine. Consequently we find in the *Vocabulario* of 1603 the earliest attempts to define concepts such as yīn and yáng, the five phases, the five depots and six palaces, and, above all, qì in a European language.

We can no longer determine to what extent, judged from our modern historical and philological viewpoint, inaccurate interpretations of the missionaries were based on a deficient understanding of the Chinese concepts by the Portuguese, by the Japanese counterparts, or both. The Chinese concept of qì (Japanese: *ki*) was described by the Portuguese as "a disposition, a quality of the thing, generally with a perjorative undertone, as in disease." They gave *xié qì* (邪气), literally "evil qì" (Japanese: *jaki*), the meaningful interpretation of "spoilt breath or pestilence." The conduits and network vessels (*jīng luò* 经络) that were never unequivocally defined in Sino-Japanese medicine

as being vessels of qì and/or blood were identified by João Ro-
drigues in his *Arte da Lingoa de Iapam* of 1604 as "veins."

The early Portuguese attempts to understand the Sino-Japanese body of knowledge concerning nature, man, and medicine
were serious.   They nevertheless failed to pave the way for a
continuing investigation of the theoretical foundation and the
language of East-Asian medicine of Chinese origin: in 1612, the
inspector Francisco Pasio forbade missionaries to acquire and apply medical knowledge; even the possession of medical literature
was no longer allowed.

With this, the first intensive, and what might have been long
and fruitful, contact between European and East Asian medicine
was interrupted out of considerations of missionary strategy. Although several decades after the missionaries had withdrawn
from medical practice in Japan, a second phase of transmission
of East Asian medical knowledge to Europe began, all subsequent transmission attempts up to the middle of the 20th century lacked consistent effort to go beyond medical practice and
penetrate Chinese medicine's own theoretical system.

2. European physicians as eyewitnesses in the Far East

The second phase of Western reception of Chinese medicine,
which was largely concerned with its practice, began in the year
1658 with the posthumous publication of a six-volume *Histo-
ria naturalis et medicae Indiae orientalis* by the Danish physician Jakob de Bondt (1581–1631). Bondt had served for a long
time in the Dutch East India Company in Batavia on Java
and through his work informed his European readers that the
Japanese treated headache, obstructions of the liver and spleen,
and pleurisy using styli of silver or steel, not much thicker than
the strings of a zither, which were inserted into the body and
made to penetrate the affected organs so that they came out
on the other side. This technique, so he claimed, he had seen
performed with his own eyes!

Whether Bondt had actually witnessed the penetration of the liver and spleen in an acupuncture treatment is not known. There is no evidence of such drastic interventions in the history of Chinese medicine. Bondt's statements were nevertheless followed quite literally 150 years later in experiments conducted in France; the inevitable catastrophic consequences of the treatment for the patients were seen by the opponents of acupuncture as tangible evidence of the harmfulness and nonsensicality of needle treatment.

In the late 17th and early 18th century, Bondt's work was followed by five other books by European eyewitnesses, including Buschof's report on gout of 1675. The *Secrets of Chinese Medicine* published in French in 1671 may have been written by one of the Jesuits who in the latter half of the 1660's was under house arrest in Canton, China. The basis for the book was, for the first time, an original Chinese text, the *Mài jué* (脉诀), an older writing of uncertain origin, possibly from the Sòng period, on pulse diagnosis.

In 1683, the Dutchman Willem ten Rhijne (1647–1700) published a *Dissertatio de arthritide: Mantissa schematica: De acupunctura* after a two-year stay from 1674 to 1676 as a station physician in the services of the Dutch East India Company. Although the Japanese authorities had forbidden the Dutch to gain any knowledge of Japanese culture, a fruitful exchange with natives nevertheless took place. Japanese doctors, for example, would visit Dutch settlements in the guise of servants in order to find out about Western medicine. Ten Rhijne questioned his colleagues and even the official interpreters about indigenous healing methods. In his comments about the practice of Japanese needle therapy, referred to for the first time by the name *acupunctura*, ten Rhine reported a broad spectrum of indications, including headache, dizziness, gray cataracts, apoplexy, rabies, epilepsy, hypochondria, melancholy, dysentery, and diseases caused by winds in the intestines. He recognized that acupuncture would remain unintelligible without the circulation system of Chinese physiology; nevertheless he never gained the opportunity to learn more about this system, or even to elucidate it for his European readers.

He summed up his observations as follows: "Cauterization and acupuncture are the two outstanding methods of the treatment of the Chinese and Japanese. They apply them to free themselves of pain. If these two peoples (and especially the Japanese) were robbed of these techniques, the sick among them would be in a miserable state, without any hope of cure or relief for their condition."

However, most writers of this time concentrated their attention not on these spectacular treatments, which were completely unknown in Europe, but rather on pulse diagnosis. Pulse diagnosis as the key to understanding the processes in the healthy or afflicted interior of the body evidently attracted the attention of Europeans much more strongly than a previously unknown opportunity to influence the interior of the body. For this reason, two further texts from this time were devoted primarily to Chinese pulse and tongue diagnosis (that is, diagnosis on the basis of changes in the coloring and surface structure of the tongue). In 1682, the German doctor Andreas Cleyer (1615–1690), after serving in the Dutch East India Company in Batavia, published in Frankfurt a collection of writings of unknown authorship under the title of *Specimen medicinae sinicae, sive opuscula medica ad mentem sinensium*, a large portion of which is a translation of the pulse text, the *Mài Jué*, but which also contained references to Chinese pharmacotherapy. The great interest in such texts is evidenced by the broad distribution of this book, which is still to be found in many libraries stocking books from this period.

The *Clavis medica ad chinarum doctrinam de pulsibus* by the Polish Jesuit Michael Boym (1612–1659), which was published posthumously in 1686, took the *Mài Jué* as the focal point and concentrated exclusively on pulse diagnosis.

In 1712, after returning from his employment in the Dutch East India Company in Japan, Engelbert Kaempfer (1651-1716) presented what was so far the most detailed description of the technique of acupuncture as regards the clinical application of the needle technique. However, he only reported on its use to treat the ominous *senki* (疝气) sickness of the Japanese, which is a generic term for afflictions of the abdominal area, including colic. Kaempfer saw the manipulation of *vapores* (vapors) in the body as the object of therapy.

It is, therefore, perhaps not surprising that as early as 1718 Lorenz Heister (1683–1758) raised the question, "why such clever nations (like the Chinese and Japanese) prized their wondrous remedies. Since this operation (acupuncture) is not used or considered to be of any use by Europeans, we do not think it necessary to describe it at length. Anyone wishing to learn about it can read the amazing descriptions given by ten Rhijne and Kaempfer." One of the people who did read ten Rhijne was Georg Stahl (1660–1734), who formed the opinion that "acupuncture served to evaporate subtle flatus with needles." The possibility inferred by advocates of acupuncture of draining off intestinal winds in patients suffering from colic by sticking needles into the intestines appeared to Stahl as proof of the capacity of individual fantasy, not as an indication of a serious therapy.

The list of books from Bondt to Kaempfer might seem impressive in retrospect, but the impact of these writings was marginal and soon disappeared. Pulse diagnosis and acupuncture triggered a transient discussion, yet none of the participants in the discussion had any reliable grasp of original Chinese knowledge. Even the Latin translations of the *Mài Jué* failed to provide illumination owing to their lack of good commentary and adequate philological skill. Hence, the debate eventually died out.

Although during the 18th century writers would again and again mention acupuncture, either to criticize it or to stimulate further research in it (for example, Gerhard van Swieten [1700–1772] in the year 1755), interest remained anecdotal. Attentive and well-read physicians knew of certain characteristics of healing in Japan and China, but the impetus was lacking to investigate them.

3. Early interpretations in electrobiology

What factors finally triggered a new wave of interest at the beginning of the 19th century are open to conjecture. The promptings by the Dutch surgeon Isaac Titsingh (fl. 1794) after his return from East Asia may have provided the external cause. Titsingh first served for 15 years in Japan in the Dutch East India Company, and after 1794 acted as the Dutch ambassador in Peking for some time.

As a doctor, Titsingh showed similar interest in the medicine of his host countries as his predecessors. Unlike other colleagues, however, he went further. He collected material evidence of the practice of Chinese medicine, including an acupuncture figure. In 1775, a Chinese merchant had by chance brought a bronze acupuncture figure with him on a visit to London, but Titsingh was the first, in his collection catalogue, to describe such a figure and present it in its medical and theoretical context, and in so doing he attracted the attention of some colleagues.

Titsingh also presented a translation of a book, allegedly of Japanese origin, about acupuncture. The sum of his promptings fell on fertile soil.

European physiologists at the beginning of the 19th century focused interest on unraveling the mystery of the supposed "divine spark," by which the living organism differed from a dead body. In this context, the 1791–1792 research by Luigi Galvani (1737–1798) in Bologna received much attention. After fierce debate especially with Allessandro Volta (1745–1827), it transpired that the electricity that Galvani had measured in the hind-legs of frogs came from the instruments used to conduct the experiments. Nevertheless, the idea of animal electricity had a lasting influence on European physiology and formed the basis for the development of electrobiology. It was inevitable that some doctors immediately presumed that the key to understanding the effects of Chinese needle therapy also lay in supposed electrical currents with the body.

France was the center of the new interest. It was here that in 1774 François Dujardin in his history of surgery had recommended the application of needles for painful parts of the body. The translation of a Japanese acupuncture book that Titsingh had introduced into the European debate gave the French physician Sarlandière the impetus to engage in a detailed investigation of acupuncture. Sarlandière in turn prompted Louis Berlioz (1776–1848), father of the composer Hector Berlioz, to conduct clinical experiments. Sarlandière was the first to experiment with the strengthening of the effect of the needle through electrical currents. Several physicians in France, Britain, Italy, and Germany followed this lead and published their findings.

One German doctor reported about the healing of two serious cases of dropsy through a combination of acupuncture and galvanism. This prompted the ministry in Berlin responsible for health care to order the effects of the therapy to be systematically examined in the Charité hospital in 1829. The report on the experiment is a protocol of terror. Two platinum needles with eyes were inserted a quarter to half an inch into the abdomen and other parts of the body. The ends of the needles were attached to the two plates of a galvanic pile.

This immediately produced in patients violent, tugging, and tearing pain, which made them scream and jerk involuntarily so that quite often the needles would fall out. The muscles closest to the insertion point contracted vigorously, a phenomenon that could most clearly be seen in the abdominal and facial muscles. Round patches of inflammation formed around the insertion points... Soon a lymph gland would appear around the first needle, bright at first, later turning dull, while the epidermis around the needle, which led to the copper pole of the pile, would rise like a blister, and on withdrawal of the

> needle would let out a kind of gas with a crack-
> ling sound.... The pulse would become larger and
> more frequent, and sometimes irregular, this latter
> phenomenon evidently being the result of the violent
> pain. The increase in vessel activity was most vigor-
> ous in the uterine system, this being the clearer the
> closer to the genitals the needles were inserted.

This description makes it understandable why subsequently all the patients in a Paris hospital rose in revolt against the application of acupuncture.

Despite the torments inflicted on test patients, participating doctors were able to announce some successes with a 24-year-old girl suffering from amenorrhea. Needling produced no success in ascites. The treatment of general dropsy "proved so terrifying that there was no thought of repeating the attempt."

Experiments to understand the effects of acupuncture and to rule out chance successes continued for half a century. In the USA, for example, the physician and chemist Franklin Bache, a grandson of Benjamin Franklin, published the findings of his ex-periments with acupuncture on prisoners suffering from rheuma-tism and neuralgia. He had come to the conclusion that the most meaningful application of the needles lay in pain relief.

The ability to reduce pain in the short or longer term is in fact probably the only point of agreement between the majority of physicians in the evaluation of acupuncture in first half of the 19th century. The publications of the research of the time offer a long list of other indications from paralysis to asphyxiation, from gout to abdominal inflammation, from early cancer to blindness. However, the arbitrary nature of the treatment pointed a dif-ferent way to each observer and permitted no standardizable conclusions.

Even in this third phase of the encounter with Chinese medi-cine, Europeans were left entirely to their own fantasies to turn the needling therapy into a sensible and reliable form of treatment. When finally a book was published under the title of *La Médecine chez les chinois* ("Medicine among the Chinese") in 1863, in which the author, Pierre Dabry de Thiersant, a former infantry officer and later French consul in China, included detailed quotations from one of the major Chinese works of acupuncture, the *Zhēn Jiǔ Dà Chéng* (针灸大成) of 1601, the "acupuncture mania" referred to by the Berlin surgeon Johannes Nepomuk Rust in his *Handbuch der Chirurgie* ("Manual of Surgery") of 1830 had already blown over. In Britain and the USA, no physician concerned for his own reputation could afford to have any truck with acupuncture for precisely the next hundred years.

Only in France did the odd few physicians keep up the interest. Their willingness to view acupuncture as an effective healing procedure was nourished mainly by reports of military physicians returning from the French colonies in Indochina, where they had observed Chinese doctors practicing needle therapy and been impressed with the apparent results.

European interest in acupuncture, to sum up this third phase of reception, was mainly concerned with its effect. Needle therapy, it seemed, was a technique, like massage or other physical healing methods, that had no theoretical basis and that deserved attention only because it at first awakened the expectation that it achieved a number of therapeutical effects by influencing recently discovered vital electrical currents in the body. Neither of these assumptions provided a long-term solid basis for its acceptance. The alleged electrical currents proved to be not so important for medicine after all, and did not provide physiologists with a definitive solution to the problem of the nature of life that was associated with interest in them, and the therapeutic effects of needle therapy remained anecdotal and unstandardizable. The developing natural sciences with their emphasis on a new approach in drug therapy and on effective surgery saw to it that only a handful of enthusiasts remained under the spell of acupuncture.

4. George Soulié de Morant and energetic acupuncture

The multivolume work *L'Acuponcture chinoise* by George Soulié de Morant, published over the period from 1939 to 1955, is also to be seen against the background of the French colonial involvement in Indochina. This work is still to this day one of the most impressive contributions of a single Western author to the explanation of the theory and the clinical applicability of acupuncture.

Soulié de Morant was born in Paris in 1879. His childhood friendship with the daughter of Théophile Gautier led him into the house of the poet, where he became acquainted with a highly educated Chinese man who taught him Mandarin. Soulié de Morant received his formal education from Jesuits, and planned to study medicine. However, the early death of his father forced him into a career that would bring earlier economic rewards. Because of his unusual knowledge of Chinese, he was sent by a bank to China, where he was soon afterwards engaged by the French diplomatic service.

Soulié de Morant remained in China until 1917. He wrote many books and essays on virtually every aspect of Chinese culture, and, as hardly any other European, gained access to the highest circles of Chinese society. It was essentially because of this that the most eminent Chinese physicians consented to instruct him in acupuncture during the twenty years of his stay. His own therapeutic achievements won him the greatest respect of his Chinese hosts, for which he received the highest civil order of the Chinese government.

After his return to France, Soulié de Morant attempted to promote acupuncture among the French medical profession. Because he was not a physician and since acupuncture had sunk to the level of an almost frivolous pursuit in the latter half of the 19th century, the immediate reaction of the medical world was one of skepticism and scorn. Against this background, Soulié de Morant considered it most helpful to publish original Chinese texts in French translation. An essay by him, published in the renowned journal *Science médicale pratique* in 1931, finally aroused the interest of two doctors, who invited Soulié de Morant to take part in collaborative research in their respective hospitals.

In 1939, the first volume of *L'Acuponcture chinoise* appeared, and in 1941, the second. Soulié de Morant sought to use available knowledge of Western medicine to understand acupuncture. However, his approach was exactly the opposite of attempts being made in China today to reduce the Chinese tradition to the essence that would allow it to be explained in terms of Western medicine (or at least not contradict Western medicine). Soulié de Morant tried to show that Western anatomy, physiology, and pathology could be interpreted anew, and could even be better understood, in terms of traditional Chinese principles.

It was probably because of this attempt to incorporate Western knowledge into the theoretical Chinese system that the publication of his book provoked a wave of hostility, which deeply hurt him personally. Soulié de Morant died shortly after completion of the third volume of his work on May 10, 1955. His collaborator for many years, the physician Thérèse Martiny, posthumously compiled volumes four and five from his notes and translations.

Soulié de Morant distinguished between different kinds of acupuncture:

> One kind is simplistic and primitive. It consists of puncturing the place of pain without considering any other knowledge. Except for conditions of recent, acute pain, such treatment gives only partial, short-term relief.
>
> Another method, somewhat better, uses points in memorized formulae. Problems are treated with little attention given to the patient or the action of the

needles; i.e., in order to tonify or disperse such and such an organ, such and a point is used; for this particular symptom, that particular point is used. This method allows moderate regulation of the organs, but does not treat the underlying cause of the problem, nor control the vital energy.

The truest form of acupuncture, which we describe here, enables the practitioner to evaluate imbalances of the vital energy, the basis of all functional illness. This is achieved above all through the study of the pulses. True acupuncture is founded on the relationship between organs, based on the circulation of energy, a system which often differs from the Western anatomical physiological model...

Noting the variations of an illness among individuals, true acupuncture from its beginning has tended to place greater emphasis on the patient. It is not the microbe that is important, but the terrain. Dr. Nakayama, a Japanese practitioner, thus states: "The illness is not the invasion itself, but the weakness that attracts the invasion."

Chinese Acupuncture, p. 3

Soulié de Morant was the first to list the effects attributed to each acupuncture point according to organs affected. These lists, unlike anything that had appeared in Chinese literature before, enabled the practitioner to apply a type of prescription acupuncture by combining points to be needled not on the basis of knowledge of the internal condition but merely on the basis of the therapeutic goals.

Soulié de Morant introduced "energy" as his interpretation and translation of the Chinese concept of qì since he was convinced that science would one day be able to demonstrate the effects of acupuncture on energetic currents within the body. Since then, most literature written for European and American

practitioners of acupuncture have interpreted the effects of the
needles in terms of energetic processes.

For the supposed pathways of qì deep in the body, Soulié
de Morant coined the term "meridian," which despite its lack
of faithfulness to the underlying Chinese concepts, has been re-
tained by nearly all authors writing for a Western public.

Under the heading of "What can acupuncture cure?" Soulié
de Morant wrote as follows:

1. First, it is advisable to point out that acupuncture can be
   used with little risk; it does not introduce poisons—foreign
   elements—into the body; nor does it conflict with any other
   treatment. In fact, it is often reported to augment the
   effect of chemical or homeopathic medicine, and dosages
   may often be reduced. The only risk in these conditions is
   the possibility of failure that leaves the patient in exactly
   the original state.

2. Lesions, defined as physical changes in part of the structure of the organism due to injury or disease, are not directly affected by acupuncture treatment. However, this
   method may temporarily reduce or nullify the pain or trou-
   ble caused by the injury.

3. Functional problems constitute the true domain of acupuncture... The meticulous observers of the Far East have suggested that except in the cases of accidents, there are no
   lesional illnesses that are not preceded by somatic, function troubles. These problems first manifest in moral and
   mental changes, so the first changes of personality constitute, in fact, the beginnings of illness. If used at this stage,
   acupuncture is most effective and is sometimes said to be
   capable of curing anything. All energetic therapies must
   be considered as first line, preventive measures which avoid
   progresssion of an illness toward a lesion which is more difficult to cure.

We should bear in mind that these lines were written in the 1920's and 30's; that is, in an age before the introduction of antibiotics. The advantages of acupuncture which Soulié de Morant had focused on would hardly awaken the interest of modern physicians for what had up to that time been an unfamiliar, exotic form of treatment.

Nevertheless, Soulié de Morant contributed greatly to paving the way for the fourth and present phase of the reception of acupuncture in the Western world. He is not responsible for this phase; the actual stimulus for contemporary enthusiasm of a section of the population for needle therapy lies in a new Zeitgeist. However, by referring to the systematic-functional approach in Chinese medicine and by being the first to interpret qì as energy, Soulié de Morant placed two catchwords in currency, which were to become quite decisive for the plausibility of the underlying theories. The fourth and present phase of reception is characterized not by the significance of the effects of acupuncture, but by the power of conviction of its theoretical background.

Finally, two further French writers, whose works have exerted considerable influence in Europe and the United States, also deserve mention here. Albert Chamfrault had already studied acupuncture before he was enlisted as a naval officer in Vietnam, where he was then able to deepen his knowledge. Between 1954 and 1969, he published a six-volume work that was devoted in particular to the implications of the qì circulation system, an aspect that Soulié de Morant had not really dealt with. Nguyen van Nghi, a Vietnamese of Chinese origin living in France, was the first Asian acupuncturist of significance for the development of needle therapy in Europe and the USA. He taught and wrote just at the time when interest in Chinese medicine and acupuncture was developing among peripheral groups and achieving general significance in health-care politics.

5. The turning point: from marginal to political

By the beginning of the 1990's, there was barely a town, let alone a city, in the Western industrialized countries without physicians or healers offering acupuncture treatment. Training courses in Chinese medical thought and practice had been developed by various societies in all European countries and the USA. One of the biggest of these in Germany is the *Deutsche Ärztegesellschaft für Akupunktur* (DÄGFA), whose courses are attended by 20,000 people each year. These figures of course do not include those who receive instruction elsewhere or who already practice acupuncture without undergoing further training.

Apart from doctors and healers who practice acupuncture in private practices, numerous hospitals have started to include acupuncture among their services. The spectrum includes special clinics with Chinese practitioners, spas offering a range of "alternative" health-care procedures, and pain clinics such as in the Grosshadern teaching hospital of Munich University's medical school. Many health insurers have found ways of covering the costs of such treatment.

This development seems paradoxical at first sight and therefore requires some explanation. In the 18th and 19th century, at a time when modern medical science was still in its beginnings, Chinese medicine failed to gain acceptance in Europe despite the vigorous efforts of numerous recognized researchers. In the latter half of the twentieth century, in competition with a highly developed, scientifically based, and in many ways outstandingly effective form of medicine, Chinese medicine is receiving such lasting affirmation from broad sectors of the population that physicians and healers are providing Chinese medical therapies, not least for economic reasons.

In actual fact, this development is not so puzzling as it seems at first sight. Some important parameters of the situation are more conducive to transcultural transfer and acceptance of Chinese healing at the end of the twentieth century than they were in past centuries.

Encouraged by colleagues in France, physicians interested in acupuncture in West Germany founded their own society in the early 1950's. It was only in the 1970's, though, that a process began whose consequences still cannot be foreseen even today. On July 26, 1971, an American journalist, James Reston, who had accompanied the US table tennis team on their historic visit to the PRC, wrote an article that appeared on the front page of the *New York Times* on how his postoperative pain had been eliminated with three acupuncture needles after an emergency appendectomy in China.

This report was played up by the whole of the Western press, and as a result the existence of China's evidently unique needle therapy, effective for reasons unknown, became a focus of public attention. Three months afterwards, a team of reputable American physicians traveled to China to observe the application of acupuncture in various hospitals. A report on the trip, which was unreservedly positive, was published in *The Journal of the American Medical Association.*

When in the following year, 1972, Richard Nixon went to China, the US President's personal physician witnessed several operations under acupuncture analgesia; on his return, he confirmed the reports of earlier doctors.

The interest of the Western world at the time was directed to the pain-relieving effects of acupuncture in surgical operations. At the beginning of the 1970's, hardly any organ of the media missed the opportunity to report on this phenomenon, most often with large colored photographs. The alleged exoticism of Chinese mentality toward coping with pain and the inscrutable, scientifically barely explicable effects of needles even in complicated surgical operations produced, against the background of decades of Chinese insularity, a blend of journalism that evidently fascinated large sectors of the public.

With the end of the Cultural Revolution and the beginning of political and economic reforms in the late 1970's, the Chinese leaders swiftly disassociated themselves from what were in reality unsatisfactory effects of surgical acupuncture analgesia (the concept of acupuncture anesthesia is completely inappropriate). With this, Western interest in this application of acupuncture disappeared. What now came into focus was the general therapeutic use of acupuncture.

Especially in the countries that had been colonially involved in East and Southeast Asia, such as the USA, Britain, France, and the Netherlands, numerous Asian immigrés who had treated patients of their own ethnic groups more or less out of public sight ventured out into the open, offering their services to local populations in general.

The first scientific studies suggested a connection between acupuncture analgesia and the effects of endogenous opioid peptides and biogenic amines in the central nervous system. This opened the possibility for serious discussion about the potential of acupuncture, even among scientists would have had to fear for their reputation if they joined debates on the movement of qì, or the existence of yīn and yáng conduits.

6. Chinese medicine in the Western world at the end of the 20th century: Interplay of market and fears

Acceptance of acupuncture in the industrialized countries of the West over the last twenty years, as would appear now, has primarily been an acceptance of the notions of the nature and appropriate treatment of illness that allegedly underlie it. Only secondarily has this acceptance rested on clinical successes. In the 1960's, certain attitudes changed among a sector of the population in Western industrialized countries. Chemistry and technology, which previously had only positive connotations, now began to lose their attractiveness, despite the fact that almost any aspect of daily life was almost unthinkable without chemistry and technology.

Regular media reports about the negative effects of chemistry on the cleanliness of air, soil, and water, on animal life, and hence on the human body and its health, as well as equally regular reports about chemical disasters in Bophal or Seveso, in Frankfurt-Hoechst, and many other places, caused chemistry to be seen in a new light, and provoked fears that extended to modern medicine. Chemical drugs come from the same factories whose products burden the environment—chemotherapy is the pride of modern medicine. It is easy to understand how the increasing detachment from the positive effects of chemistry were associated with a sense of alienation from a form of medicine that had closely relied on chemistry.

The same process of change is seen in attitudes toward technology. The impact of technology on daily life, once celebrated in world exhibitions as the solution to the millennia-old problems of humanity, now came to have a pale aftertaste for a certain section of the population. Technology is felt by many to destroy nature and also to destroy relationships between human beings. The picture of the railroad and freeway is no longer associated principally with communication between distant regions; it is equated with the carving up of stretches of land once intact.

Technology, and not least nuclear technology, is viewed as a threat, and this evaluation is carried over to medicine, whose whole pride rests on the application of technology in diagnosis and therapy. Technical diagnosis, though, can provoke fear and drive a wedge between patient and doctor. Many patients have the feeling that inexorably neutral machinery produces the diagnosis and informs the doctor with paper printouts or computer images. These patients wonder whether the dominance of technology in these areas allows any room for the perception of individual distress.

The advertising for Chinese medicine focuses precisely on these fears. The fuzzy concept of "natural healing," which in actual fact is barely applicable to Chinese medicine, offers an impression of security that their bodies will not be polluted with chemicals and suggests that the personal application of the needles guarantees a traditional doctor-patient relationship with the promise of sympathy and empathy. The diagnosis of inspection, listening and smelling, inquiry and pulse-taking aims to evaluate the suffering of the individual, not to compare the patient with standard values, any deviation from which is *a priori* considered morbid.

Important for the success of acupuncture and Chinese medicine has been the notion of qì. Acupuncture and Chinese medicine became attractive and plausible in Western countries overnight when shortage in oil supplies from the oil-producing countries in the 1970's made the Western world aware of the energy problem. Since those years, energy supply has come to be the most important existential problem of the industrial nations of the West. Securing energy supplies has repeatedly led to international conflicts culminating in military action. Domestic energy policy and the controversy about the best forms of energy for the future have led to violent squabbles in national politics. Even for the private household, concern about availability and affordability of energy since the energy crisis of the 1970's is not to be underestimated.

Against this backcloth, "Chinese healing," as interpreted by Western writers, at least serves to solve the issue of the energy problem within the individual's own body. By explaining disease in terms of energetic disturbances, Chinese medicine gains plausibility, but a plausibility that arises out of conceptual adaptation to Western fears, not out of the historical reality of Chinese thinking.

A further conceptual adaptation to the concerns of a section of the population enhances the attractiveness of Chinese medicine. Many metaphors of killing, defense and attack, which have become prevalent since the 19th century with the development of bacteriology and more recently in the realm of popular descriptions of immunology, have been taken for granted in China since ancient times. This brand of figurative use of language, however, does not appear in the version of Chinese medicine propagated in the West.

For the population of Europe increasingly disquieted by the threat of war, reports about the latest developments in immunity research in Western medicine presents a picture of war in the body in often quite drastic metaphors. The mass media report on "daily massacres, frightful carnage, and secret acts of sabotage," "hidden allies and the search for wonder weapons" in the battles between killer cells, and viruses, and so forth, on the one hand and antibodies supported by biochemistry and surgery on the other.

This kind of war reporting from the inner life of the body is understandable to some and frightening to others. Anyone afflicted by disease seeking rest and harmony finds it hard to come to terms with the fact that modern drugs are engaged in a belligerent struggle to destroy the enemy in the organism. Largely as a result of ruthless TV reporting, the general public is aware of unavoidable undesired side-effects on the civil population in real war, just as it is aware of the side-effects of drastic chemotherapy.

In contrast to reports from the battlefield of modern immunology, the theory of Chinese medicine freed of its martial metaphors gives the impression that it can lead patients back to the harmony of the great whole. It offers solace where modern medicine offers only the uncertainty of a murderous battle.

Quite a few patients experience modern medicine as a supermarket of possibilities, in which many specialists each investigate the organism from their narrow angle and recommend appropriate remedies based on their narrow view. The loss of a central authority guiding the patient toward an existentially meaningful understanding of his or her illness parallels the loss of "central meaning" within society in general. In daily life, a lack of central meaning, though enjoyed by those who are able to take full advantage of individual freedom, is bothersome for the many who find life hard to cope with and need guidance. Similarly, if modern medicine, which as any form of medicine is a reflection of the spirit of the times, fails to offer many patients any deep, innermost reason for their suffering—at least, this is what a certain sector of the population feels.

The systematic-functional approach of Chinese medicine fills this gap. Of the heterogeneous mixture of different approaches that have arisen over the past two thousand years, the only approach to have found its way to the West is the one that appears to have been neglected by modern medicine or, to put it more accurately, one which is taken for granted in modern medicine at a theoretical level, but which neither the general practitioner nor the specialist appears to be able to put into practice, and which for the patient might as well not exist at all.

The systematic approach in Chinese medicine and hence also in acupuncture interprets the body as a unity and the individual organism as a part of the whole universe. Chinese natural philosophy appears as an attractive alternative at a time when many people, consciously or unconsciously, suffer from the lack of reference to a whole, and are unable and unwilling to experience the whole in explanation models offered by the traditional churches. The notions of yīn and yáng and the five evolutive phases suggest answers to many questions and solutions to many problems that seem pressing today without having to resort to conventional religions.

The notions of the necessary harmony between man and his environment on the larger scale, and between the individual functional spheres of the body on a smaller scale address the doubts of many who cannot escape the impression that traditional politics and theology are either unable to adequately deal with the threats to future life or actually actively encourage the catastrophes in store.

The systematic and at the same time nonmetaphysical approach of Chinese medicine, with regard to both the individual body and the universe, answers the needs of these people and has its primary justification in these needs.

Nonetheless, this attractive systematic approach is only a child of our times. It has secured for Chinese medicine and acupuncture a certain amount of popularity because it addresses the existential needs of a sector of the population at the end of the 20th century. The coincidence between the systematic approach and the existential needs has provided an initial push that has brought acupuncture into the limelight, yet for acupuncture to gain long-term recognition and avoid homeopathy's fate of being the eternal outsider, it requires substantiation, which in our Western civilization means the stamp of approval of science.

For a large proportion of users of acupuncture, it is of course of no direct consequence whether the application of acupuncture achieves scientifically demonstrable effects. The systematic approach is attractive because a preliminary cure for a wounded soul is achieved through its integration in a system of ideas that gives meaning to an individual illness, that traces the problems of the head or back, skin or mouth to an underlying cause in the body, and that relates, if necessary, the underlying cause in the body in turn to an underlying cause in the existential environment of the patient.

Given the multiple morbidity that ails our society in the eyes of a growing section of the population, it is reassuring to know that there exists an explanatory model at least for the multiple morbidity in the body that is capable of pinpointing the central problem and perhaps even of treating it. The fact that this central problem is expressed in unusual terms such as "kidney yáng depletion" lessens fears, since such terms evidently cannot be construed as referring to biochemical or biophysical disturbances, which would have to be treated with chemical or technical methods that have increasingly fallen into discredit. Concepts such as kidney yáng depletion refer to a deviation from an equilibrium in the great world plan that can be reversed.

All these factors alone might be reason enough for Chinese medicine—even if it only fits this description in part—to be viewed as a meaningful complement, if not an alternative, to conventional Western medicine. It should also be added that, in contrast to the unsuccessful efforts in the 18th and 19th centuries, Chinese medicine in China has now come to be recognized as a lucrative export product, and in the Western commercial world is seen as a profitable investment.

It is particularly from this side (i.e., from the commercial world) that idealizing reports with cliché-coining titles such as "Healing from the Far East" are promoted in large-circulation magazines. This kind of reporting generates continuing interest among patients who originally may have had no affinity with such therapies, but who as a result of negative experiences in their dealings with contemporary biomedicine or as a result of unsatisfactory treatment in the past are now willing to give an allegedly Chinese alternative a chance.

The short air flights that have drawn Europe and America closer to China have brought more and more visitors into contact with Chinese medicine on its home ground. Chinese tourist managers have developed routines to show foreign travelers Chinese medicine in practice, especially Chinese drug therapy, which was hitherto only of marginal interest in the West, but which, for economic reasons, is a more viable export product. Tourists are given free diagnoses, which inevitably end with therapeutic suggestions. A considerable turnover is generated in this way. To what extent the medicines provided contain admixtures of highly effective substances from modern medicine not declared on the labels can scarcely be evaluated. The effects achieved cause many to seek Chinese medical health care on their return.

7. The spectrum of supply

Not all, but most of the books on acupuncture written for MD and non-MD students of acupuncture and general lay-audiences in Western countries place the systematic-functional approach of Chinese medicine in the foreground. They begin with an explanation of the doctrines of yīn and yáng and the five phases with lists of their correspondences. They show the system of the

supposed meridians that for two thousand years provided the
basis of needle therapy. The meridian system illustrates the way
in which the functional spheres of the body are interlinked, providing a graphic representation of the holistic view of Chinese
medicine.

In this way, Western literature presents those elements of
Chinese medicine that have a chance of providing a conceptual alternative to contemporary biomedicine and a complemen-
tary method of treatment. It would be impossible for Chinese
medicine to be brought to the West in its entirety or in some
purely original Chinese form. First, there is no Chinese medicine
as a finished, closed healing system. Chinese medicine developed
dynamically over two millennia much as medicine in the West
did from its Hippocratic beginnings around the 500 B.C. The
development of Chinese medicine within the framework of its
traditional theoretical system came to a standstill long before
the end of the cultural environment that made this medicine
possible and made its conceptual basis plausible. None of the
major areas—theory, acupuncture, and pharmacy—have undergone any significant innovation since the beginning of the 17th
century.

In particular, acupuncture, after a peak that was reached with
the publication of the "Great Encyclopedia of Acupuncture and
Moxibustion" (针灸大成 zhēn jiǔ dà chéng) in 1601, gradually
degenerated to a folk medicine, prompting the famous physician
Xú Dàchūn (徐大椿, 1693-1771) in a detailed survey published
in 1754 to speak of the "loss of a tradition" and the nonexistence
of able acupuncture practitioners. In 1822, the Chinese government classed acupuncture as a method of treatment that learned
men should not be exposed to and forbade the imperial medical
college to instruct students in its practice.

Against this background, the question arises as to what "Chinese medicine" should be transmitted to the West. The practices and theoretical conceptions that in the political climate
of the People's Republic of China have been chosen from the

heterogeneous heritage as meaningful? The varied practice free of political influence, based on personal interpretation of traditional opinion and techniques among representatives of Chinese, for example, on Taiwan? The pragmatic approach relatively free of theory that is widespread in Japan? Or any of the various Chinese approaches of the last two millennia? In trying to answer this question, one problem lies in the fact that there is no criterion for judging any one of these approaches in relation to another. They all have their effects. Practitioners of each of them can point to satisfied patients. Failure is of course also common to all.

Time and time again, each practitioner sees the astounding effect of the needles, but no explanatory model that would convince and completely satisfy at least a majority of practitioners is in sight. So far, the scientific approach to acupuncture has not followed satisfactory methodologies. Studies producing negative conclusions have no influence over practice, since such evaluations strengthen the conviction of those who would deny science the right to judge procedures whose conceptual basis lies outside scientific thought structures.

In this context, we should also consider the difficulties faced by medical faculties of universities confronted with demands to introduce Chinese medicine into the curriculum. Neither the theoretical basis, diagnosis or even the theory of Chinese medicine can be standardized. Graduates of modern medicine, even though they may later attain different levels of proficiency as physicians, have at least all had roughly the same training to the highest possible contemporary standards and have proven their knowledge through officially supervised examinations. This is not possible in Chinese medicine.

A medicine school or faculty that decides to include acupuncture in its curriculum has no criteria for the selection of teaching staff. If it has the idea to take on Chinese practitioners, it must decide first of all if preference is to be given to traditional practitioners who have no university education, who have learned their skills through self-study or a long teacher-student relationship, and who practice "classical" Chinese medicine, or to graduates from modern teaching institutions in the People's Republic of China who are trained to varying degrees in Western medicine, but who are no longer capable of practicing traditional medicine uninfluenced by modern anatomical, physiological, and pathological ideas.

Whichever option a medical school chooses, there are no objective criteria for evaluating the knowledge of prospective teachers in either group. Students attending one clinic in southern Germany are astounded to hear the therapies there are not spoken of flatteringly in another clinic in southern Germany, and vice versa. The reason for this is that the doctors in the one come from Peking, whereas those in the other are from Shanghai. Each group practices its own version of "Chinese medicine," and denies the other version any legitimacy even though it has no empirical or scientific grounds for doing so. The fact that these clinics are subject to no state or technical quality control is only one of the many ramifications of this situation.

Quite apart from the absence of an objective method of finding a skilled doctor in one or another group, the medical school, should it have reached the conviction that it has found a suitable candidate, cannot, given the nature of Chinese tradition, be sure that the candidate will be willing to pass on all his knowledge. Secret knowledge, to which only the mastermind has access, is still an important part of the prestige of an outstanding doctor in China. Even today, the best doctors refuse to pass on all of their knowledge either in medical colleges or to individual students assigned to them.

If the administration gives preference to Westerners, there would be a large number of different groups to choose from, most of which contest each other's competence. There are groups who, without any scientific evidence, say that getting the feeling of qì (得气 *dé qì*) at the needle insertion point is the *conditio sine qua non* for the effectiveness of acupuncture treatment; other groups maintain precisely the opposite. There are groups who regard a strong electrical impulse as a prerequisite for successful treatment (which raises the question as to how acupuncture could have survived for two millennia without artificial electricity), while other groups of equally successful acupuncturists produce their effect through shallow needling whereby the needles penetrate the skin barely a millimeter. There are groups who state, again without any scientific proof, that acupuncture can only produce effects when ancient Chinese notions are followed, and these fundamentalists formulate their allegedly classical notions in a way that the ancient Chinese could not even have heard of. Other groups would rather discard all ancient Chinese concepts, believing that acupuncture's legitimacy can only be based on modern neurological or endocrinological theories.

It is not possible to make a reasonable choice from this plethora of options. Wherever a choice has been made, it has rested on local availability and personal recommendations. The students taught by such staff cannot be sure what quality of training they are getting since the chances are that in the nearest medical bookstore they will pick up a "standard work" of acupuncture that represents a completely different approach, or that they will come across an introduction to Chinese medicine whose terminology follows a completely different system of interpretation, translation, or transcription from the one to which they are accustomed. In either case, they will be confused. The same insecurity also affects patients.

The impossibility of objectively determining which of the old or modern approaches is the best and of standardizing this approach in theory and clinical practice is of course only one of the difficulties facing attempts not only to transfer Chinese medicine to the West, but also to anchor it in the Western academic framework. A second difficulty is closely related to this one, and is often overlooked. Irrespective of whether Western supporters of Chinese medicine take their notions of Chinese medicine from the older or more recent history of Chinese medicine, however hard they devise a purely Chinese alternative to Western medicine, they always fail because of the difference in attitude between Chinese and Western traditions to the stringency of thought systems.

The Western preference for thought systems that are free of internal contradictions and that constitute truth until a new truth provides better explanations with fewer contradictions is diametrically opposed to an East Asian tradition that judges thought systems by how well they prove themselves to be in practice rather than by how true they are. The yīn-yáng and five-phases doctrines are in many respects mutually exclusive, as when, for example, one assumes the existence of six and the other the existence of five depots in the body. The Western solution to the problem, which is to open the body and see whether there are five or six organs, stands in contrast to the Chinese tendency to reckon with six organs in the yīn-yáng doctrine and with five organs in the five-phase doctrine.

The yīn-yáng doctrine is legitimized by its being a logical system of correspondence and by proving itself capable of evaluating and influencing numerous processes in the body and hence in the human organism. The five-phase doctrine is legitimate for precisely the same reason: it too is logically derived from the notion of systematic correspondence and proves itself by being capable of evaluating and influencing numerous processes in the body and hence in the human organism. Consequently, traditional Chinese medicine bases itself on both doctrines, and sees no contradiction between them.

Another example is offered by pulse diagnosis. For those who are still capable of thinking in purely traditional categories, the various schemes for feeling the wrist pulse that are presented in ancient literature represent no contradiction. The physician has the choice of either feeling the pulse with three fingers or with one finger. Using three fingers, light pressure with the index finger above the imaginary line level with the styloid process allows him to feel the state of the lung and heart, greater pressure with the middle finger on the imaginary line enables him to feel the state of the spleen, and greater pressure still with the ring finger allows him to feel the liver and the kidney, which similarly lie in the depths of the body. Also in accordance with the doctrines of correspondence the physician can apply a little pressure to feel the lung and heart, a little more pressure to feel the spleen, and still greater pressure to feel the liver and kidney. According to a third (and certainly not the last) variant, he can, with one finger, apply a pressure equal to the weight of three beans to feel the lung, a pressure of six beans to feel the heart, a pressure of nine beans to feel the spleen, a pressure of twelve beans to feel the liver, and finally a pressure that brings the fingertip almost to the bone, to feel the kidney.

All three procedures are logically justified in themselves, since they are all based on systematic correspondence. Nevertheless, they go against Western thinking, which in the face of a "this-as-well-as-that" framework naturally poses the "is-it-this-or-that?" question. Authors writing for a Western public have no choice but to answer the "is-it-this-or-that?" question with regard to the number of organs, the pulse diagnosis schemes, and many other details.

Consequently, in all descriptions of Chinese medicine written for Western users, what is perhaps the only real alternative that Chinese medicine offers in comparison with Western thinking is adapted to the usual patterns of, precisely, Western thought. When one further considers the fact that the Western variant of Chinese medicine, by explaining the central concept of qì as energy and by selecting only those elements from the heterogeneous tradition that do not appear obsolete or scientifically absurd, is divorced from the original Chinese tradition, then it is easy to understand that the reception of Chinese medicine is not a mechanical, but a creative act, whose further development is conditioned more by the expectations and demands of a Western population than by the marshalling of scientific evidence.

Chronological Table

ca. 16th–11th century B.C.	Shāng
1045?–256 B.C.	Zhōu
722–481 B.C.	Chūnqiū (Spring and Autumn) Period
403–221 B.C.	Zhànguó (Warring States) Period
221–206 B.C.	Qín
206–A.D. 220	Hàn
206 B.C.–A.D. 8	Early (Western) Hàn
9–23	Wáng Máng Interregnum
25–220	Eastern (Late) Hàn
220–581	Liùcháo (Six Dynasties) Period
221–265	Sānguó (Three States) Period
265–316	Western Jìn
317–420	Eastern Jìn
420–589 (386–581)	Southern and Northern Dynasties
581–618	Suí
618–907	Táng
907–960	Five Dynasties
960–1279	Sòng
960–1126	Northern Sòng
1127–1275	Northern Sòng
907/946–1125	Liáo (Kitan)
1032–1227	Xīxià
1115–1234	Jīn (Nüzhen)
1279-1368	Yuán (Mongol)
1368–1644	Míng
1644–1911	Qīng (Manchu)
since 1911	Republic of China
since 1949	People's Republic of China

SELECT BIBLIOGRAPHY

1. History

R. Croizier, *Traditional Medicine in Modern China*, Cambridge, MA: Harvard University Press, 1968.

D. Harper, *Early Chinese Medical Literature: The Mawangdui Medical Manuscripts*, London: Kegan Paul, 1997.

G.E. Henderson and M.S. Cohen, *The Chinese Hospital: A Socialist Work*, Unit. New Haven: Yale University Press, 1984.

M. Kubny, *Qi: Lebenskraftkonzepte in China; Definitionen, Theorien und Grundlagen*, Heidelberg: Haug Verlag, 1995.

Lu Gweidjen and J. Needlham, *Celestial Lancets: A History and Rationale of Acupuncture*, Cambridge: Oxford University Press, 1980.

W. Michel, *Willem ten Rhijne und die japanische Medizin (II)*, Studien zur deutschen und französischen Literatur, 1990, 40, 57-103.

W. Michel, *Frühe westliche Beobachtungen zur Moxibustion und Akupunktur*, Sudhoffs Archiv 77 (1993), 195-222.

W. Michel, *Engelbert Kaempfer und die Medizin in Japan.* In: Detlev Haberland (hsg.) Engelbert Kaempfer: Werk und Wirkung. Stuttgart: Franz-Steiner Verlag, 1993.

T. Ots, *Medizin und Heilung in China: Annäherungen an die traditionelle chinesische Medizin*, Berlin: Dietrich Reimer Verlag, 1995. 2 Auflage.

V. Scheid, *Beobachtungen zur Verbindung von chinesischer Medizin und Biomedizin in der Volksrepublik China*, ChinaMed 1994, 4, 16-22.

V. Scheid, *Meister, Lehrlinge, Lehrer und Studenten: Zur Wissensvermittlung in der chinesischen Medizin*, ChinaMed 1995, 5, 38–44.

P.U. Unschuld, *Medicine in China: A History of Pharmaceutics*, Berkeley, Los Angeles, London: University of California Press, 1986.

P.U. Unschuld, *Medicine in China: A History of Ideas*, Berkeley, Los Angeles, London: University of California Press, 1985.

P.U. Unschuld, *Nan-Ching: The Classic of Difficult Issues*, Berkeley, Los Angeles, London: University of California Press, 1986.

P.U. Unschuld, *Huichun: Chinesische Heilkunde in historischen Objekten und Bildern*, Munich: Prestel, 1995.

2. Variants of reception

D. Bensky and A. Gamble, *Chinese Herbal Medicine: Materia Medica*, Seattle: Eastland Press, 1986.

F. Friedl, *Arzneimitteltherapie,* Das neue China, 1986 13, 18-20.

Michael Hammes and Thomas Ots, *33 Fallbeispiele zur Akupunktur aus der VR China: Ein klinisches Kompendium*, Stuttgart: Hippokrates-Verlag, 1996.

Joseph M. Helms, *Acupuncture Energetics: A Clinical Approach for Physicians*, Berkeley, CA: Medical Acupuncture Publishers, 1995.

Eric Marié, *Grand formulaire de pharmacopée chinoise*, Vitré: Editions Paracelse, 1991.

M. Porkert, *The Theoretical Foundations of Chinese Medicine*, MIT Press, Cambridge, MA: 1974.

M. Porkert, *Klinische Chinesische Pharmakologie*, Heidelberg: Verlag für Medizin Dr. Ewald Fischer, 1978.

M. Porkert, *Lehrbuch der chinesischen Diagnostik*, Heidelberg: Verlag für Medizin Dr. Ewald Fischer, 1976.

G. Soulié de Morant, *Chinese Acupuncture*, English edition edited by Paul Zmiewski, Brookline, MA: Paradigm Publications, 1994.

E.A. Stöger, *Arzneibuch der chinesischen Medizin*, Stuttgart: Deutscher Apotheker Verlag, 1995.

G. Stux, N. Stiller, R. Pothmann, A. Jayasuriya, *Akupunktur: Lehrbuch und Atlas*, Heidelberg–New York–Tokyo: Springer Verlag, 1985.

3. A Chinese view

Cheng Xinnong, *Chinese Acupuncture and Moxibustion*, Peking: Foreign Language Press, 1987.

Index